Praise for *The Diabetes Miracle*

"Inspiring. . . . If you're worried about diabetes and want to find out how it can be tackled, Diane's story could be well worth a read."
—*Healthy Magazine*

"Diane Kress, a registered dietitian, sets out a three-step program . . . your doctor is the best resource for medical and dietary concerns, but this book can be a helpful supplement."   —*Washington Post*

"A guide to understanding diabetes as well as a plan for managing it . . . A thorough examination of diabetes and its management for those who are ready to take control of their own health."
—Technorati.com

"Easy to understand and implement, the lifestyle program outlined by Diane Kress could be a step in bringing down the shocking national numbers of those facing type 2 diabetes."   —*Tucson Citizen*

ALSO BY DIANE KRESS

The Metabolism Miracle Cookbook

The Metabolism Miracle

THE
DIABETES
MIRACLE

3 Simple Steps
to Prevent and Control Diabetes
and Regain Your Health . . . Permanently

DIANE KRESS, RD, CDE

Da Capo
LIFE
LONG
A MEMBER OF THE PERSEUS BOOKS GROUP

Cataloging-in-Publication data for this book is available from the Library of Congress.
First Da Capo Press edition 2011
First Da Capo Press paperback edition 2013

ISBN 978-0-7382-1505-1 (hardcover)
ISBN 978-0-7382-1540-2 (e-book)
ISBN 978-0-7382-1601-0 (paperback)

Published by Da Capo Press
A Member of the Perseus Books Group
www.dacapopress.com

Note: This book is intended only as an informative guide for those wishing to know more about health issues. In no way is this book intended to replace, countermand, or conflict with the advice given to you by your own physician. The ultimate decision concerning care should be made between you and your doctor. We strongly recommend you follow his or her advice. Information in this book is general and is offered with no guarantees on the part of the authors or Da Capo Press. The authors and publisher disclaim all liability in connection with the use of this book.

Da Capo Press books are available at special discounts for bulk purchases in the U.S. by corporations, institutions, and other organizations. For more information, please contact the Special Markets Department at the Perseus Books Group, 2300 Chestnut Street, Suite 200, Philadelphia, PA, 19103, or call (800) 810–4145, ext. 5000, or e-mail special.markets@perseusbooks.com.

10 9 8 7 6 5 4 3 2 1

Dedicated to those who seek
the knowledge, support, and empowerment
to best care for their own health and the health
of those who are dear to them.

Contents

PART TWO

The Diabetes Miracle Plan:
Rest, Reset, and Retrain the Pancreas

PART THREE

The Diabetes Miracle Lifestyle

Introduction

If you were to randomly stop Anyone on Any Street in Anytown, USA, and ask the following three questions, I'm certain that the answer to at least one of the questions would be *yes*:

1. Do you have a grandparent, parent, or sibling who has diabetes?
2. Do you have a friend or coworker who has diabetes?
3. Does your husband, wife, or anyone in your extended family (cousins, aunts, uncles) have diabetes?

Almost everyone knows someone with prediabetes or type 2 diabetes, and the numbers are rising on a daily basis. Every nineteen seconds someone is diagnosed with diabetes.

Although we most often associate an epidemic with a fast-spreading disease, such as the flu, the term *epidemic* has been linked to type 2 diabetes since early this century. In December 2006, the International Diabetes Foundation (IDF) published data indicating the enormity of the diabetes epidemic. Since the IDF's alarming report, there has been tremendous worldwide attention regarding the implications of this uncontrolled global epidemic.

Understanding Met B, Prediabetes, and Type 1 and 2 Diabetes

METABOLISM B

Also known as metabolic syndrome, Met B appears to be rooted in a genetic predisposition to insulin imbalance and insulin resistance. This hormonal imbalance appears to be triggered by a combination of physical, emotional, or environmental stressors and progressively leads to escalating weight, LDL cholesterol, triglycerides, blood pressure, and blood sugar. Without proper diet and exercise, Met B can lead to prediabetes and type 2 diabetes.

PREDIABETES

Prediabetes is a metabolic condition that occurs when fasting blood glucose is elevated but not to the degree of type 2 diabetes levels. Diagnosis of prediabetes is made when lab-drawn fasting blood glucose is 100–125 mg/dL* or hemoglobin A1C is 5.7–6.4. Although prediabetes is considered to be reversible, without intervention (e.g., positive changes in diet, exercise, and maintenance of a healthy weight), it is likely to lead to irreversible type 2 diabetes in ten years or less.

DIABETES

Type 1: Type 1 diabetes is an autoimmune disorder with possible environmental triggers, such as a virus or environmental toxins. It accounts for between 5 and 10 percent of cases of diagnosed diabetes. Once known as juvenile diabetes or insulin-dependent diabetes, type 1 diabetes is most commonly diagnosed in children and young adults—although anyone can develop type 1 diabetes. It is a chronic disease in which the pancreas produces little or no insulin. An outside source of insulin is required for life. There is currently no cure of type 1 diabetes.

Type 2: Type 2 diabetes is a metabolic disorder that is the result of genetic factors and lifestyle stressors (obesity, overweight, age, poor diet, lack of exercise, emotional stress). It is by far the most prevalent type of diabetes, with almost 95 percent of diagnosed cases of diabetes being this type. It is

---

*Outside the United States, glucose is usually reported in units of mmol/L (millimoles per liter). One mmol/L = 18 mg/dL. To convert mg/dL to mmol/L, divide by 18 or multiply by 0.055.

diagnosed when lab-drawn fasting blood glucose exceeds 125mg/dL or hemoglobin A1C exceeds 6.4. Although it occurs mainly in adults, children also can be diagnosed with type 2 diabetes. A progressive disease that is the result of insulin resistance and relative insulin deficiency, type 2 diabetes can be treated with any of the following: diet/exercise, diet/exercise/oral medications, or diet/exercise/insulin.

In the United States today, one in ten adults has diabetes. A whopping 104.8 million Americans have either prediabetes or type 2 diabetes. According to the American Diabetes Association (ADA), seven million Americans are unaware that they have diabetes. In 2010, the Centers for Disease Control and Prevention (CDC) warned that by the year 2050, as many as one in three adults in the United States could have diabetes.

Type 2 diabetes is not only a concern of adults; obesity and overweight are also taking their toll on children. According to the American Heart Association (AHA), approximately 4.5 percent of children were overweight between 1963 and 1970. Today, approximately 17 percent of children and adolescents aged 2 to 19 are obese. Since 1980, obesity prevalence among children and adolescents has almost tripled, and one in three children is now considered overweight or obese.

Diabetes is also a worldwide problem. According to World Health Organization (WHO) estimates, by 2025, 300 million of the world's population will be affected by diabetes.

WHY DIABETES? WHY NOW?

What is going on? Why has the incidence of diabetes risen so dramatically—and why is the diagnosis rate expected to continue to rise?

Six factors are combining to accelerate the diabetes epidemic in the United States and around the world:

1. Baby boomers (people born between 1945 and 1964) make up a large percentage of the American population. The incidence of type 2 diabetes increases with age, and Americans are becoming an older population.

2. We're living longer. Advances in diabetes management, including the development of various medications, are enabling people with a diagnosis of diabetes to live longer.

3. Diabetes is being diagnosed at younger ages. Earlier diagnosis is expanding the number of people under the umbrella of prediabetes and type 2.

4. Minority populations that currently have a higher rate of diabetes are increasing.

5. We are consuming diets of increased portion sizes of carbohydrate-dense foods. Restaurant portions of pasta, rice, fries, as well as supersized soft drinks, bagels, muffins, pretzels, burger buns, and ice creams are sometimes three to four times larger than they were twenty years ago.

6. People are less physically active and are becoming more sedentary. In place of walking, we rely on cars to take us everywhere. Instead of physically playing, children are spending more time passively watching television, using computers, playing video games, texting, talking on the phone, and listening to their MP3s. Appliances have taken the activity component out of our home lives, while longer workdays have taken away from exercise time. The majority of jobs are no longer physical in nature; they involve largely sedentary office work, customer service, computers, or desk jobs.

A combination of these factors has lead to the burgeoning epidemic that is exponentially gaining strength.

THE COSTS OF DIABETES

Having type 2 diabetes is one thing. Having type 2 diabetes under control is another. A person whose diabetes is under good control can prevent or greatly forestall diabetic health complications. On the other hand, a person with diabetes that is out of control over a long period of time will systematically chip away irreversibly at his long term health. These complications can include:

HEART DISEASE AND STROKE

- Adults with diabetes have heart disease death rates about two to four times higher than adults without diabetes.
- The risk for stroke is two to four times higher among people with diabetes.
- In 2005–2008, of adults aged 20 years or older with self-reported diabetes, 67 percent had blood pressure greater than or equal to 140/90 mmHg or used prescription medications for hypertension.

BLINDNESS

- Diabetes is the leading cause of new cases of blindness among adults aged 20–74 years.

KIDNEY DISEASE

- Diabetes is the leading cause of kidney failure, accounting for 44 percent of new cases in 2008.
- In 2008, a total of 202,290 people in the United States with end-stage kidney disease due to diabetes were living on chronic dialysis or required a kidney transplant.

NERVOUS SYSTEM DISEASE (NEUROPATHY)

- About 60 to 70 percent of people with diabetes have mild to severe forms of nervous system damage.

AMPUTATION

- More than 60 percent of non-traumatic lower-limb amputations occur in people with diabetes.
- In 2006, about 65,700 non-traumatic lower-limb amputations were performed in people with diabetes.

After adjusting for population, age, and sex differences, average medical expenses among people with diagnosed diabetes were 2.3 times higher than expenditures would be in the absence of diabetes. The total cost of diagnosed diabetes in the United States in 2007 was $174 billion. With the additional costs of undiagnosed diabetes, prediabetes, and gestational diabetes, the total cost of diabetes in the United States in 2007 is $218 billion! According to the CDC, the number of Americans with diabetes is projected to double or triple by 2050.

Based on the dire predictions for the future health of the world regarding obesity and diabetes, it is imperative to slow this trend drastically by making the right lifestyle changes with diet and exercise. The correct style of diet coupled with increased physical activity can actually reduce the risk of diabetes. Keep in mind that the statistics regarding the future incidence of diabetes are based upon the assumptions that the increases in new cases of diabetes will continue at the present rate and that we will continue to treat (or mistreat) diabetes as it is being treated now.

WHAT THIS BOOK WILL DO FOR YOU

You may be trying to make sense of this confusing, overwhelming, and often frustrating disease. Perhaps you seek to prevent it, control it, or live better with it. Maybe someone in your family has been diagnosed with diabetes, or you want to protect your friends and family from developing diabetes.

If you have prediabetes and you make the recommended changes in your lifestyle that are outlined in *The Diabetes Miracle*, you can actually prevent the onset of type 2 diabetes. If you have type 2 diabetes, you will absolutely improve its control. You may be able to prevent, decrease, or even eliminate the need for medications. This book can enable you to finally understand prediabetes and type 2 diabetes in such an intimate way that its control will become second nature, empowering you to live a healthy, unfettered life with ease and confidence.

The Diabetes Miracle is your guide to learning everything about preventing or controlling type 2 diabetes. It provides priceless, easy-to-understand information that you can use or pass along to your family and friends. It will empower you to reach your goals. Person by person, family by family, we can make the right choices to stop this epidemic. I am hopeful that forty years from now, we will look back to this time in medical history and say that it was the high point of the incidence of diabetes. I hope that we will be able to say that from 2011 on, the incidence of uncontrolled type 2 diabetes began to decrease across the generations, and we are all healthier because of the informed choices we made.

The right tools make even the most complex job easier. Now, *The Diabetes Miracle* will give you the tools for successful diabetes management: getting your blood sugar under control quickly, efficiently, and naturally. There is no such thing as uncontrollable type 2 diabetes—there is only diabetes that is not yet controlled. This book will give you the tools to get your prediabetes or type 2 diabetes under control and to keep it that way for the rest of your healthy life.

I am thrilled to have the opportunity to write this book. As a person with type 2 diabetes, I've faced the need to understand a condition that will be part of the rest of my life. There is no cure for type 2 diabetes. No surgery can erase it; no amount of weight loss takes it away. But, type 2 diabetes is *always* controllable, and *The Diabetes Miracle* will show you how.

PART ONE
DIABETES MADE SIMPLE

RETHINKING DIABETES:
A REVOLUTIONARY NEW APPROACH

Would you call it a miracle if you found yourself physically, mentally, and emotionally healthier than you can remember? Would it be a miracle if in your middle age, you actually looked and felt better than you did when you were younger? How would you feel if your blood tests came back in the normal range with the use of little or no medication? What about finally losing that stubborn excess weight and keeping it off? Wouldn't it be incredible to wake up feeling refreshed and you had energy to spare until bedtime? Wouldn't it be great to sleep through the night? Until now, the preceding "miracles" were unlikely for those with diabetes. But when you follow *The Diabetes Miracle*, they can be expected.

Because of the Diabetes Miracle way of life, I no longer hold my breath at the doctor's office when my blood is drawn, silently praying that my lab results did not worsen since my last checkup. When I awaken each morning, I don't experience that sinking feeling as I wait the five seconds for my fasting blood sugar to register. I no longer own a pill box filled with my daily ration of prescription medications that "band-aided" some very serious medical conditions. I don't cringe when the seasons change because this season's clothes may no longer

BLOOD SUGAR TARGETS

Personal blood sugar targets for home glucose monitoring, the number of daily tests, and the timing of these tests should be set by your physician or health care provider. Remember to ask your MD for your own personal targets at your next office visit.

The following are examples of my personal blood sugar targets:

Fasting: My personal blood sugar target upon waking in the morning: 70–120 mg/dL.

After a meal: My personal blood sugar target timed two hours after the start time of any meal: 140 mg/dL or less.

fit me. I don't panic from a high blood sugar reading of 190 two hours after my "prescribed" dinner—I know how to immediately bring it down to normal AND can figure out what caused that unusual spike.

I feel very free. Why? Because after creating and following the Diabetes Miracle lifestyle, I have achieved my personal desired weight, and my lab work remains pristine with no medications for diabetes, hypertension, or cholesterol. Daily blood glucose monitoring gives me continual proof that my diabetes is under control. Complications from diabetes are not part of my personal vocabulary—I don't have them.

It wasn't always this way. I had always been conscientious with diet and exercise. When I began to feel poorly and had unexplained weight gain despite my healthy lifestyle, I shifted my academic focus to nutrition and eventually became a registered dietitian. When I was diagnosed with type 2 diabetes, I didn't even realize that I was a person "at risk." In fact, I was directing the nutrition component of a diabetes center! As a certified diabetes educator and a registered dietitian, I was not only teaching but also dutifully following the dietary guidelines prescribed by the American Diabetes Association and accepted by the American Dietetic Association and American Medical Association

(AMA). I was only 38 when I was diagnosed, but in retrospect, it was clear that I was headed toward type 2 diabetes since the age of 21.

In my early twenties, I noticed a small roll around my middle that no amount of dieting and exercising helped. I felt my energy ebb, I had aches and pains, and my focus and concentration began to decrease. I became moody and irritable. My periods were heavy and irregular. I became so interested in health, diet, and exercise that I switched my major to nutrition. I followed a low calorie, low-fat, low-cholesterol lifestyle with regular exercise.

As the years passed, although strictly adhering to my diet, my weight continued to increase. My once-low blood pressure began a slow rise to normal levels, then to borderline high, then to full blown hypertension. My low cholesterol readings began to rise even though I followed the prescribed diet and ate no red meat or saturated fat. My two children were born each weighing more than nine pounds. At the time of their birth, my physician did not yet routinely screen for gestational diabetes, yet it is clear that I had gestational diabetes during both pregnancies. It took more than five years to get pregnant between my daughter and my son. I now understand that an increased rate of miscarriages and fertility issues are linked to blood sugar fluctuations.

Between the ages of 21 and 38, I slowly but surely gained weight. It didn't matter if I ate or didn't eat, if I exercised or didn't exercise. No matter what I did, my weight marched on, a puffy, bloated weight that defied my textbook healthy lifestyle.

Then, at the age of 38, at work at the diabetes center that I nutritionally managed, I sat at my desk thinking: "I'm so thirsty." "All I do is run to the bathroom." "I'm so tired." Then it hit me. These were textbook statements of someone who has diabetes. I got out a blood glucose monitor and checked my blood sugar right then and there. It was over 200. I couldn't believe it. I went to the bathroom, rewashed my hands, and did the test again, with the same result.

That week I saw my internist and had fasting lab work done—twice. I was diabetic, my lipids (fats including triglycerides and cholesterol) were elevated, and my blood pressure was elevated. I was 38 and left the office with enough prescriptions to wallpaper a small room. And all this happened when I was a relatively young woman and lived a supposedly healthy lifestyle.

THE TRADITIONAL APPROACH TO TREATING DIABETES

The traditional ADA diabetes diet plan was based on calories and contained approximately 50–55 percent carbohydrates, approximately 20–25 percent protein, and the remainder in fat. Calorie requirement was determined based on gender, age, height, desired weight, and activity level. I was eating three carbohydrate-based meals and a bedtime snack. I was following and teaching the "carb is a carb" philosophy of the ADA, meaning that as long as my daily intake of carbohydrates fell within the amount I was required to consume at a meal, it didn't matter what type of carb I chose to eat.

It's amazing when I think of it now, but two of my three meals (breakfast and lunch) required that I *increase* my carbohydrate intake to meet my "carb requirement." I obediently did. The ADA diet booklet we supplied to all patients contained pages of carb suggestions, including full strength fruit juice, cookies, fries, regular gelatin, and so on. This was a pretty easy pill to swallow—however, it also required that I swallow some very real pills to control my blood sugar. After years of adhering to the program verbatim and teaching it to hundreds of people who were newly diagnosed with type 2 diabetes, I began to see a trend: There was no significant long-term improvement in most people's weight, blood sugar, cholesterol, triglycerides, blood pressure, depression, fatigue, aches/pains, problems in focus and concentration, or carb cravings from this program—my own experience included.

Time and time again over the upcoming months and years, my patients would regain their initial marginal weight loss and require increasing types and doses of medications to barely control their rising blood sugar, cholesterol, blood pressure, and even depression. They followed their diet and exercise protocol, but they never saw lasting improvement.

I should mention that there is a saying in the diabetes community that goes like this: *If you are lucky enough to live long enough with type 2 diabetes, you will require insulin.* This is because most medications for diabetes increase pancreas fatigue and, eventually, diet, exercise, and oral medications are not enough to control blood sugar. Once oral medications stop working, insulin is the last resort. And in the past, it was practically a given that a person with diabetes would eventually require insulin injections.

As a diabetes educator and a person living with type 2 diabetes, it became clear that something was wrong with the program we were dispensing to treat diabetes. I began to look at diabetes from a "root perspective." I went back to the basics and asked the questions: how and why did this disease-process begin, and what was causing it to worsen over time? Must diabetes be a "runaway train" with the last stop requiring either a pillbox filled with medications, or insulin? Could something be done with lifestyle to stop the progression and enhance health?

I'm thrilled to report that after years of research and thousands of successful patients, the Diabetes Miracle became a reality. The Diabetes Miracle is a lifestyle guide designed for the millions who have Metabolism B or are already diagnosed with prediabetes or type 2 diabetes (see definitions of these terms on page x).

For the first time, a diet and exercise protocol, a lifestyle, is available that gets to the root of Metabolism B as it rests and rehabilitates the overworked endocrine system, reprograms the pancreas/liver combination, and finally enables good health and well-being with as little medication as possible. I live the Diabetes Miracle way of life, as do hundreds of thousands around the globe. And now you can, too.

UNDERSTANDING TYPE 1
VERSUS TYPE 2 DIABETES

If you are reading this book, there is a good chance that you (or someone you know and love) have a diagnosis of prediabetes or type 2 diabetes. The diagnosis may be new, or it may be something you've lived
with for many years, but it's a good bet that you feel confused, frustrated, or even defeated by this disease. Part of the problem and cause
for confusion is that until very recently, the medical community had
not fully understood the process and progressive path to type 2 diabetes.

Unlike type 1 diabetes, an autoimmune disease in which the immune system destroys the insulin-producing beta cells in the pancreas
and causes a relative absence of insulin, those with type 2 diabetes
usually spend many years silently overproducing insulin caused by an
overactive pancreas. The two types of diabetes may share a name, but
they are very different.

Unfortunately, from a dietary perspective, type 1 and type 2 diabetes
have been treated as "diabetes" although the conditions are close to
being opposites in physiology. People with type 1 do not have any significant insulin response to a rise in blood sugar, whereas those with
type 2 diabetes overrespond to a rise in blood sugar by releasing excess
insulin. The two types of diabetes are not the same, but because of the
blanket approach that was brought to diabetes treatment and management, there has been a mishmash of contradictory information, mass
confusion, poor blood sugar control, and frustration. So let's make this
clear: *The Diabetes Miracle* is written to the specific needs of individuals with type 2 diabetes.

The Diabetes Miracle is not only based on the latest research but is
also a fresh way to view, understand, and manage each of the *progressive* stages that can lead to type 2 diabetes: uncontrolled Metabolism B,
prediabetes, and type 2 diabetes. This book will help you to understand
how it's possible to progress (or have progressed) from normal blood
sugar levels to type 2 diabetes. Most important, it offers a very different

and proven diet and lifestyle program for getting diabetes under control and keeping it under control for a lifetime. With *The Diabetes Miracle*, you will become expert on the disease, how and why it occurred, how to manage it, and how to become healthier because of it.

A PROGRESSIVE DISEASE

Until recently, a person was considered to be either diabetic or not diabetic, similar to being pregnant or not pregnant. Now we realize that a person is "on the road to diabetes" for years before type 2 diabetes is diagnosed.

The first stage is uncontrolled Metabolism B, a genetic condition that predisposes a person to insulin imbalance. If left untreated, uncontrolled Met B can lead to a compilation of progressively worsening medical conditions, including overweight; hypertension; and elevated LDL cholesterol, triglycerides, and blood sugar. The symptoms of Met B begin silently and over a period of years; the pancreas's overreaction to blood sugar with excess insulin contributes to excess fat deposits in the blood and on the body. Enlarged fat cells develop misshapen insulin receptors that lead to insulin resistance. Insulin resistance means that even though excess insulin is present, it does not "fit" the cell doors, and sugar begins to build in the bloodstream.

If this fat-gain stage is not recognized and controlled, Met B can progress to prediabetes, a condition in which the overfed and oversized fat cells become even more resistant to insulin. The pancreas continues to overrelease insulin and blood sugar (unable to enter cells) begins to rise. If prediabetes is not managed, it can advance to type 2 diabetes, an irreversible disease in which the pancreas no longer produces adequate insulin, insulin resistance worsens, and glucose can build to dangerous levels in the blood.

In fact, it is now accepted that if you become aware of your uncontrolled Met B or prediabetes and make the right lifestyle changes, you might actually *reverse* the progression and prevent the development of type 2 diabetes. In this book, you will learn to identify Met B through your own lab work, family history, and daily symptoms.

If you have already progressed to type 2 diabetes, you will learn to control it through lifestyle and manage it with much less or no medication.

THE EXCHANGE LISTS FOR MEAL PLANNING—AND WHY THEY DON'T WORK

There have been dietary programs to treat diabetes for more than sixty years. So why not use traditional programs to control prediabetes or to manage type 2 diabetes? After all, the ADA developed the "Exchange Lists for Meal Planning" in the 1950s.

Well, sixty years ago in the spectrum of diabetes management is the Stone Ages of diabetes. Because so little was known then about this metabolic disease, the methods used to treat it were rudimentary at best. The Exchange Lists were devised and used long before self-monitoring of blood sugar even existed. They were inflexible, confusing, difficult to follow when eating combination foods or dining out, and may have actually helped speed the progression from prediabetes to type 2 diabetes.

It wasn't until the 1950s that the first oral diabetes medications were released. We now know that these initial medications forced the already overworking pancreas to work harder. Yes, they squeezed the pancreas to release more insulin—although it was already overreleasing insulin. The initial oral medications actually fatigued the pancreas faster.

Believe it or not, the Exchange Lists are still taught for diabetes control. The Exchange List diet is based on calories with approximately 50–55 percent of the calories coming from carbohydrate foods. (Note that carbohydrate is the main nutrient people with diabetes have difficulty processing, and 100 percent of carbohydrates turn into blood sugar.) The Exchange List diet dictates the number of servings of particular groups of carbohydrates that are "allowed" at each meal or snack along with the precise ounces of protein and teaspoons of fat for each meal or snack. A typical meal plan looks like this:

2 servings of starch
1 serving of fruit
1 serving of milk
2 ounces of meat
1 serving of fat.

There is little room for diversity, the lists make eating out very diffi-cult, eating combination foods close to impossible, and the diet does not really help improve blood sugar. If you were never able to gain con-trol of your diabetes using Exchange Lists, it is totally understandable!

The Exchange Lists stayed rigidly in place until the 1980s, when the ADA released a radical diet change in a concept called "Carbohydrate Counting." Carb-counting diets are also based on calories, and 50–55 percent of these calories come from carbs. The big change was that in-stead of dictating the particular group of carbohydrates "allowed" at a meal or snack, the patient was taught that "a carb is a carb." This meant that as long as the carb grams were equal, you could consider 15 carb grams from an apple = 15 carb grams of white bread = 15 carb grams of jelly beans = 15 carb grams of ice cream = 15 carb grams of lentils.

Although these foods are very different in nutrition and type of carb content, they are viewed as interchangeable. There is no regard to the glycemic index (the speed at which carbs change to blood sugar). In the 1980s, the ADA promoted the idea that the type of carb you chose didn't matter as long as the carb grams were within your target range. So quick, high-glycemic (high impact on blood sugar) carbs and slower, low-glycemic (low impact on blood sugar) carbs were considered inter-changeable. In fact, the Exchange List book now included brownies, regular jelly, sugar, honey, and more. As you can imagine, the carb-counting diet did not work to slow the progression to diabetes or to allow a person to get good blood sugar control because it remained 50–55 percent carbs without regard to the glycemic index or the dietary fiber content of foods. A slice of whole-wheat bread with its high-fiber content was considered the same as a slice of white bread with no fiber content because their carbohydrate content was the same.

In the mid-1990s, the ADA recommended that 50–70 percent of calories could come from carbohydrates in the diet for diabetes. This was an attempt to lower the fat content in diets. The assumption was that fat was making people gain weight and have high blood lipids and blood pressure. It is now abundantly clear that the higher the percentage of carbohydrates in the diet, the higher the resultant blood sugar, the faster the pancreas fatigues, and the more out of control is the progression to type 2 diabetes.

In 2004, the ADA diet was back to recommending about 50–55 percent carbs. In a 2004 study published in the journal *Diabetes*, participants were given either the ADA-recommended moderately high–carb diet with a carbohydrate:protein:fat ratio of 55:15:30, or a low-carb diet with a carbohydrate:protein:fat ratio of 20:30:50. The mean twenty-four–hour serum blood sugar at the end of the ADA high-carb diet was 198 mg/dL. The mean twenty-four–hour serum blood sugar at the end of the low-carb diet was 126 mg/dL. This indicates a drop of 36 percent in mean serum blood sugar as compared with the higher-carb diet over the course of the study.*

As of today, the ADA is taking a seemingly noncommittal position regarding diet for diabetes. "Tailor the diet to the person." "Emphasize the difference between low– and high–glycemic index carbs." "There is no defined amount of carbohydrate to recommend to patients with

---

Diabetes 53 (2004): 2375–2382.

diabetes." "Work the foods a person prefers to eat into their meal plan." "Choose foods from all the food groups." Although the ADA has recognized that a lower-carb diet produces improved blood sugar readings, it has not endorsed it as a matter of course.

How Diabetes Miracle Is Different

After more than thirty years of work as a specialist in type 2 diabetes, weight reduction, and metabolic syndrome, I developed the scientifically based and world-renowned program known as *The Metabolism Miracle*. This program's diet precepts are at the heart of proven weight loss and improved health and well-being for everyone with Met B, prediabetes, and type 2 diabetes. In *The Diabetes Miracle*, these proven techniques are fine-tuned exclusively for those with type 2 diabetes. The diet is the heart, and all the easy-to-understand information on diabetes is the soul of this book.

Not based on calories, traditional carb counting, or exchange lists, *The Diabetes Miracle* is based on three necessary sequential steps:

1. carb detox,
2. carb rehab, and
3. carb-balanced maintenance.

The type, amount, and timing of carbohydrates are all equally important. In addition, physical activity (not Olympic-grade, but increased movement of muscles) works in conjunction with diet to quickly stop the runaway train.

The Diabetes Miracle program has three steps. Step 1 consists of eight weeks of a purposely "lower"-carb diet to rest and rehab the overworked pancreas. Step 1 will also be your base diet and includes liberal amounts of neutral foods, such as lean protein, heart-healthy fats, and vegetables, with the option of a 5 gram carb choice at all meals and bedtime. Step 2 consists of eight-plus weeks of all the base foods from Step 1 PLUS the addition of delicious, gentle carb choices, in the right amount, at the right time. In essence, you sprinkle healthy carbs throughout your entire day and into the night in addition to your base neutral foods. When you reach your desired weight, and your blood sugar, blood pressure, and other labs are normal on as little medication as possible, you will live on Step 3. The clear-cut diet guidelines in *The Diabetes Miracle* begin to work within the first few days, with improved blood sugar readings before week's end. With *The Diabetes Miracle*, you can expect to:

- Really, truly understand type 2 diabetes for the first time;
- Understand the potential complications of uncontrolled diabetes and how to prevent them;
- Stop the progression from Met B to prediabetes, prediabetes to diabetes, or gain control of type 2 diabetes on an easy, livable program;
- Lose weight and keep it off. The majority of weight loss will be targeted around your middle, love handles, and excess back fat;
- Have increased energy, sleep great, look younger, and feel healthier;
- Get the best blood sugar readings you have experienced since your diagnosis on the least amount of (or no) medication;
- Improve your blood pressure, LDL cholesterol, HDL cholesterol, Hb A1C, triglycerides, and vitamin D level;
- Learn about your medications and about monitoring blood sugar;
- Learn the special tweaks necessary for exercising with diabetes; and
- Learn how a positive mind-set can actually improve your blood sugar.

It's time to close the door on confusion, fear, frustration, and failure when it comes to blood sugar control. *The Diabetes Miracle* will give you the key to health and well-being as well as a brand new lease on life. Let's get started . . .

WHAT IS DIABETES?

The most common type of diabetes is type 2 diabetes. It accounts for 90–95 percent of cases and usually develops in adults. Type 2 was once known as adult-onset diabetes or noninsulin-dependent diabetes, but it is important to note that children can be diagnosed with type 2 and that many people with this form of diabetes use insulin to help control their blood sugar.

Type 2 diabetes has two main components: insulin resistance in inadequate production of insulin. Insulin resistance means your pancreas may be producing plenty of insulin, maybe even an excess amount, but your cells become resistant to the effects of insulin—the hormone that regulates the movement of sugar into your cells. Another component of type 2 diabetes is that after years of overproducing insulin, the pancreas fatigues and no longer produces enough insulin to maintain a normal glucose level.

There's no cure for type 2 diabetes, but you can manage—or even prevent—the condition. Managing starts with eating healthy foods, exercising, and maintaining a healthy weight. If diet and exercise aren't enough, you may need diabetes medications or insulin therapy to manage your blood sugar.

In the human body, the preferred random glucose level for the brain and body runs between 65–139mg/dL. In normal metabolism, with the help of the pancreatic hormones insulin and glucagon, blood sugar is almost always within this range. It does not matter if the person eats or doesn't, overeats or doesn't eat enough—normal hormonal regulation keeps the blood sugar in the healthy range.

In the case of someone with prediabetes, daily random blood sugar can vacillate from under 65 to as high as 199mg/dL (after eating). When someone has type 2 diabetes, blood sugar can exceed 200mg/dL. Hormonal regulation is skewed, and as a result, the octane of the blood is often out of the normal range. If unchecked, high blood sugar can lead to a host of health problems with potentially serious repercussions, including diseases of the eye (including retinopathy and cataracts), kidney disease (nephropathy), nerve damage (neuropathy), circulatory and vascular disease, as well as heart disease (effects of high lipids and blood pressure).

WHAT ARE THE TYPES OF DIABETES?

You may have heard people say they have diabetes, but do you know which kind? In addition to the red-flag zone of prediabetes, there are three very different types of diabetes.

PREDIABETES

Prediabetes is diagnosed when your blood glucose levels begin to venture out of the normal zone. Prediabetes brings an elevation of fasting blood sugar to 100–125 mg/dL. When you have a diagnosis of prediabetes, that means you're on the fast track to developing type 2 diabetes unless you take steps to reverse it. Think of the diagnosis of prediabetes as a blessing: You still have the opportunity to stop the progression to type 2 diabetes, which is irreversible. Although it is known that diabetes can be prevented or delayed among adults at high risk through modest weight loss and increased physical activity, a study published in the April 2010 issue of the *American Journal of Preventive Medicine* revealed that only half of American adults with prediabetes reported attempts to lose weight or exercise more in the past year.

GESTATIONAL DIABETES

If you are a man, you will never develop gestational diabetes. Gestational diabetes mellitus (GDM) is unique to women who develop this temporary diabetes as a result of pregnancy. In most cases, the mother's blood sugar returns to normal after childbirth. This condition occurs in about 5 percent of all pregnancies and is usually diagnosed by blood tests between the twenty-fourth and twenty-eighth week of the pregnancy. There are approximately 200,000 cases of gestational diabetes in the United States each year.

If a woman is diagnosed with gestational diabetes, she should be instructed about proper diet and blood glucose testing. If her blood sugar is not brought into the normal range for pregnancy despite diet and medically cleared physical activity, the most common choice of medication is insulin injection. If GDM is not controlled, the baby is almost always born weighing more than nine pounds (he was "overfed" glucose in utero) and may develop hypoglycemia upon delivery. The child may also be prone to type 2 diabetes later in his life.

If a woman has a diagnosis of type 2 diabetes prior to her pregnancy, she cannot also have gestational diabetes. A woman who has type 2 diabetes before her pregnancy has type 2 diabetes during her pregnancy. In addition, women who have had GDM have a greater chance of developing type 2 diabetes later in life. According to the CDC, half of women who had gestational diabetes will develop type 2 diabetes during their lifetime. If you have a diagnosis of GDM, you should have your fasting blood glucose checked annually.

TYPE 1 DIABETES

Between 5 and 10 percent of people with diabetes have type 1 diabetes, thought to be the result of an autoimmune disorder that renders the pancreas incapable of producing insulin. *The Diabetes Miracle* is written specifically for those with type 2 diabetes, a genetically based metabolic disorder in which the pancreas continues to make insulin, but it is ineffective or produced in an insufficient amount.

TYPE 2 DIABETES

The most common form of diabetes by far is type 2. Previously known as adult-onset diabetes, it is now on the increase in children as well as adults. The condition can take years to develop and results from a combination of inadequate insulin production as well as increasing insulin resistance (rendering insulin less effective). As of 2005, 104.8 million Americans had either prediabetes or type 2 diabetes (more than 25 percent of the U.S. population). Type 2 diabetes is fairly evenly split between men and women, according to the ADA.

Type 2 is thought to be a product of genetics and lifestyle factors or stressors. Some of the most common lifestyle factors or stressors include increased weight; decreased activity; emotional stress; physical stress including pain, illness, and surgery or recovery from surgery; and a carb-dense diet for those genetically predisposed to insulin imbalance.

Even at diagnosis, most people with type 2 diabetes already have some degree of elevated cholesterol, triglycerides, blood pressure, and midline fat. More than 55 percent of people initially diagnosed with type 2 diabetes are overweight.

Type 2 diabetes is more common in African Americans, Latinos, Native Americans, Asian Americans, and Pacific Islanders. The risk of onset increases with age. There is presently no cure for type 2 diabetes, but it is a controllable disease with the aid of diet, medication, and exercise as needed to keep blood sugar in the normal zone.

The Diabetes Miracle is designed for those with Metabolism B, pre-diabetes, or type 2 diabetes.

YOUR BODY, BLOOD SUGAR, AND MORE

We derive energy for all the body's processes from the food we consume. Although we hear so much about the calories in the food we eat, food contains macronutrients (carbohydrate, protein, fat), vitamins, minerals, antioxidants, and fiber.

Of the three major nutrients found in food (carbohydrate, protein, and fat), only one has a tremendous impact on blood sugar: carbohydrate. Less than 50 percent of ingested protein turns to blood sugar and at a very slow rate of conversion. Less than 10 percent of fat turns to blood sugar and at an even slower rate of conversion. But 100 percent of carbohydrate turns to blood sugar, and the conversion begins within minutes of ingestion.* Some examples of carbohydrate foods that cause a rise in blood sugar are bread, rice, pasta, crackers, cereal, potatoes, fruit, milk, yogurt, legumes, desserts, and chips.

When carbohydrate is consumed, it causes blood sugar to rise. This rise in blood glucose causes the brain to send a signal to the pancreas to release the hormone insulin. The pancreas is a glandular organ containing beta cells that produce and secrete insulin. It is located behind the stomach (in the area below your left breast). The pancreas also produces other hormones (glucagon, somatostatin, and amylin) and enzymes that help regulate blood sugar and digest foods.

I like to envision the hormone insulin as a key. After a meal, when carbohydrate causes blood sugar to rise, insulin is released. Insulin keys enter the blood stream and attach themselves to keyhole-like receptor sites on muscle and fat cells. The insulin key must match the

---

*In *The Diabetes Miracle*, I will refer to blood sugar and blood glucose interchangeably.

cell's keyhole. Insulin can then unlock the muscle or fat cells and allow blood sugar to enter these opened cells. Muscle cells will then use the sugar for energy, whereas fat cells become storage sites for future fuel needs. Note that insulin and insulin receptors must match to enable the fit that allows the key to open the door to the cell.

When a person has type 2 diabetes, his pancreas has been overproducing and overreleasing insulin in response to rising blood sugar for years. Because of years of excess insulin production, excess insulin keys have been opening excess fat cells. This explains why people with prediabetes often have excess fat on the outside (midline roll of fat) and on the inside (elevated cholesterol and triglycerides) as well as have the potential to develop a fatty liver.

The fatter the fat cells become, the larger they become. As fat cells stretch, their keyholes change shape. Over time, the connection of the insulin keys to the receptor sites begins to fail. Compare it to putting your front-door key in your back-door lock—the key is there, but it doesn't fit, and the door can't open.

As time goes by, the pancreas begins to fatigue from excess insulin production. It is making plenty of keys, but they don't fit, and the brain continues to call upon the overworked pancreas to produce still more insulin. The pancreas will eventually begin to fatigue. The situation now includes misshapen and stretched out insulin receptors along with a fatiguing pancreas. This scenario eventually results in inadequate insulin production and insulin that no longer fits receptors. As a result of this progressive process, prediabetes becomes irreversible type 2 diabetes.

If you have diabetes, it means that your pancreas has experienced some degree of fatigue. The degree of pancreas fatigue and insulin resistance determines if you have:

- prediabetes
- type 2 diabetes that responds to treatment with diet and exercise

- type 2 diabetes that responds to treatment with diet/exercise and oral medication
- type 2 diabetes that requires treatment with diet, exercise, and insulin.

Depending on how many years you have had uncontrolled prediabetes or diabetes, and the severity of your insulin imbalance, you are probably experiencing both of the following scenarios by the time you are diagnosed:

Decreased insulin production: The insulin-making beta cells in your pancreas may no longer be capable of producing enough insulin to open the right amount of cells to normalize your blood sugar.

Increased insulin resistance: After years of overfeeding fat cells with excess blood sugar, the connection between your insulin and insulin receptors has become impaired. Some say that fat cells have stretched and so, too, have the receptors. As a result, the lesser amounts of insulin that are now released don't perfectly fit the insulin receptors.

As a result of a decreased amount of insulin production and increased insulin resistance, blood sugar backs up in the bloodstream. The brain continues to send signals to the pancreas to release more insulin; the cells are not being opened and therefore are not receiving the sugar. Ironically, a person with prediabetes or type 2 diabetes usually has higher than normal levels of blood sugar AND insulin in their bloodstream at the same time.

Type 2 diabetes is a progressive, genetically mediated metabolic malady that results from progressive fatiguing of the pancreas, decreased insulin production, and resistance to insulin. The good news is that although type 2 diabetes is not reversible, it can be controlled with proper diet, exercise, and medication (if necessary).

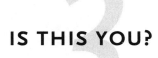

IS THIS YOU?

As mentioned previously, there are several conditions that put you at risk for developing diabetes. Some are not in your control (age, family history, or race); others are within your ability to change (overweight, inadequate exercise). Knowing what puts you in the danger zone for diabetes can help you to understand what you can do to better manage any predisposition toward type 2 diabetes or type 2 diabetes itself.

PERSONAL RISK FACTORS FOR DIABETES

The following is a list of factors that increase your risk of developing type 2 diabetes:

- Prediabetes (fasting blood sugar: 100–125mg/dL, HbA1C: 5.7–6.4)
- Age: over 45 years of age
- Family history of diabetes
- Overweight
- Sedentary lifestyle with no regular exercise
- Aberrations in lipid panel: high total cholesterol, LDL cholesterol, triglycerides, low HDL cholesterol
- Hypertension

- Certain racial and ethnic groups (e.g., non-Hispanic blacks, Hispanics/Latino Americans, Asian Americans and Pacific Islanders, and American Indians and Alaska Natives)
- Gestational diabetes, or having a baby weighing close to 9 pounds or more at birth
- Diagnosis of polycystic ovarian syndrome (PCOS)
- Certain fertility issues or history of miscarriage.

BARBARA

Barbara has nearly all the risk factors for developing type 2 diabetes. You will see that her story is not out of the ordinary (risk factors are mentioned parenthetically):

Barbara, a 55-year-old (age) African American (race) woman, is overweight and inactive (sedentary lifestyle). Her mother had type 2 diabetes (family history) and died before age 60 of a heart attack (the leading cause of death among diabetics).

Barbara had years of PCOS (common with Met B), with irregular periods, bad cramps, and heavy bleeding. After several miscarriages and difficulty with fertility (fertility issues) she finally became pregnant. At week 28, her routine blood screening produced a diagnosis of gestational diabetes (linked to insulin imbalance). Her son, Ray, was born at 9 pounds, 6 ounces (GDM and having a baby born weighing more than 9 pounds).

At the age of 48, after years of heavy menstrual bleeding and a diagnosis of ovarian cysts (linked to insulin imbalance), Barbara had a hysterectomy.

She currently takes medication for hypertension, high cholesterol, and elevated triglycerides (metabolic syndrome). Her last physical exam showed her fasting glucose at 116mg/dL (prediabetes).

Barbara's profile shows that she has a myriad of risk factors for type 2 diabetes. Following the Diabetes Miracle lifestyle program might actually prevent her from developing type 2. However, without taking the proper steps, it's only a matter of time before Barbara progresses to type 2 diabetes, which is irreversible.

THE TRADITIONAL SYMPTOMS OF DIABETES

You have probably seen a list of the traditional symptoms of type 2 diabetes on pamphlets, public service commercials, posters in your doctor's office, on the news, and in magazines. Although they may be familiar to some, many of you may think to yourself when you see them, "That's just not me!"

The traditional symptoms include:

- excessive thirst
- frequent urination
- increased hunger
- blurry vision
- frequent infections
- wounds that won't easily heal.

It should be noted that when a person is regularly experiencing these symptoms, they may be experiencing blood sugar that is regularly over 200mg/dL. Diabetes is diagnosed when fasting blood sugar exceeds 125mg/dL. By the time a person experiences such symptoms as extreme thirst, ravenous hunger, and frequent urination, he has probably had type 2 diabetes for quite some time.

Because the onset of type 2 diabetes is usually quiet and takes years to develop, many endocrinologists routinely add six years to a person's diagnosis date if there is no previous lab work to determine when blood sugar crossed the line from normal to prediabetes to diabetes. With this frame of reference, if you were diagnosed with type 2 diabetes as a result of lab work drawn at age 56, these specialists would assume you possibly had diabetes since age 50 and simply weren't aware of it.

QUIET SYMPTOMS OF DIABETES

During the years preceding a definitive diagnosis, if a person listens—*really* listens to his body—he will hear diabetes whispering in his ear. The following is a list of symptoms that are not always associated with diabetes but actually are very common in the lives of those folks who eventually are diagnosed with type 2 diabetes:

FATIGUE

The fatigue caused by fluctuating blood sugar is not the same as fatigue caused by lack of sleep or physical overexertion. Blood sugar–based fatigue can occur first thing in the morning upon awakening from sleep. Blood sugar fatigue is also common after meals (within two hours of eating). This unique form of fatigue feels as if you have run out of steam, are drained, and need a pick-me-up (caffeine or a snack). The fatigue from fluctuating blood sugar causes sluggish movement and thought and suppresses motivation and enthusiasm.

CARB CRAVINGS

The track of normal blood sugar is a smooth curve, with a gradual rise that lasts about two hours from the start of a meal, seamlessly followed by a slow, smooth decline back to the normal blood glucose range within about four to five hours after the start of the meal. When insulin is imbalanced and blood sugar is contorted into peaks and valleys, it feels more like riding a wild rollercoaster. Many people with diabetes can literally feel their blood sugar swings. They regularly report feeling extremely tired, fiercely hungry, unable to think clearly, shaky, and slightly nauseous.

Almost immediately after eating carbohydrates, people with diabetes instantaneously, albeit temporarily, feel much better. Unfortunately, this peaceful feeling does not last long; within a few short hours, the symptoms return. The rise and fall of blood sugar with the accompanying blood sugar peaks and valleys can be temporarily abated by eating carbohydrate foods. The quick, temporary fix that people with diabetes get from carbohydrates can turn into a carb addiction. Unfortunately, excess carb intake gets the pancreas working overtime. The more fatigued the pancreas becomes, the greater the impact on blood sugar, and the stronger the addiction to and cravings for carbohydrates.

MILD DEPRESSION

For many years before you are diagnosed with diabetes, your pancreas produces excess insulin. Excess insulin causes drops in blood sugar. Living with lower than normal blood sugar is like running a car on the wrong octane gas. When blood sugar is low, the brain is not fueled properly and cannot optimally perform its many tasks. The symptoms of vacillating blood sugar may mimic the symptoms of mild depression. It's possible that many people who have been diagnosed with mild depression are actually people with uncontrolled Met B, prediabetes, or type 2 diabetes. If that is the case, it might help to explain why many "depressed" people get little relief or actually feel worse on antidepressants instead of feeling a lift and improved clarity, purpose, and energy.

ANXIETY, IRRITABILITY, AND A SHORT FUSE

As the diabetes train moves down the tracks, the person begins to experience an increase in high blood sugar readings, with high readings replacing low blood sugar readings throughout the course of a day. The feelings of anxiety; nervousness; and "coming out of your skin"; along with such physical symptoms as rapid heartbeat, cold sweat, tightness in the chest, difficulty swallowing, and shallow breathing all can be symptoms of the anxiety caused by high blood sugar. There is some indication that panic attacks can be precipitated by blood sugar swings.

POOR SHORT-TERM MEMORY AND INABILITY TO FOCUS

Blood sugar fluctuation causes inappropriate glucose levels in the brain. When blood sugar is either too low or too high, the brain is not receiving the proper strength of fuel. A person cannot properly process and store information if her brain is without proper fuel. As a result, you may have difficulty remembering where you left your keys, why you walked into that room, and how to balance your checkbook as well as retaining what's being taught in class.

MIDLINE FAT DEPOSITS

The pancreas is located deep inside the abdominal cavity, between the stomach and the spine. The adult pancreas is about six to seven inches in length. Part is located behind the stomach, and the other part fits in a curve of the small intestine. To get an idea where this important gland resides, make the OK sign with your right hand (touching the tip of your thumb to the tip of your index finger. Keep the remaining three fingers straight). Place your hand in the center of your belly, just underneath your lower ribs, and point the three fingers to the left. Your hand is approximately at the level of the pancreas.

The OK sign exercise is significant because it shows you the area where the pancreas first releases insulin. The first fat cells that have the opportunity to connect with the insulin are in the area closest to the pancreas. Hence, fat deposits accumulate around the middle; belly fat, love handles, back fat, and muffin top are pronounced in those with insulin resistance caused by uncontrolled Met B. Excess insulin contributes to a person becoming apple-shaped rather than pear-shaped.

APPLES AND PEARS

An apple-shaped person holds most of his fat in his midsection: belly fat, love handles, back fat, chest/breast area. A pear-shaped person has most of her fat in the hips, buttocks, and thighs. For years, we've heard that it is heart-healthier to be a pear rather than an apple. You can now see why that is true. Those who are apple-shaped most likely have Met B. People with Met B progressively develop midline fat, hypertension, high cholesterol and triglycerides, and high blood sugar. This package of symptoms (metabolic syndrome) is what causes the high incidence of heart disease, cardiovascular disease, and stroke and can ultimately lead to type 2 diabetes. You cannot change your body type because you cannot change your type of metabolism, but you can control your insulin and therefore control the amount of fat on your body and in your bloodstream.

VERY EASY WEIGHT GAIN/DIFFICULT WEIGHT LOSS

A person who has uncontrolled Met B responds to rises in blood sugar with excess fat-gain hormone: insulin. (A person with normal metabolism responds to blood sugar with the correct amount of insulin.) If both individuals count every calorie they consume and account for every calorie they burn through exercise, they will **not** achieve the same fat loss. The person with uncontrolled Met B will respond to every gram of carbohydrate and every rise in blood sugar with excess insulin release and will find it difficult to lose fat despite counting every calorie and every exercise moment.

DIFFICULTY FALLING OR STAYING ASLEEP

Blood sugar is the main fuel source for the body. For the most part, blood sugar remains in the normal range of 70–120 mg/dL. The highest blood sugar readings in normal metabolism would reach a maximum of 139 mg/dL two hours after the start of a meal.

If blood sugar is elevated, it is probable that you will have difficulty falling and staying asleep. Blood sugar out of the normal range does not

SLEEP APNEA AND PREDIABETES/ TYPE 2 DIABETES MAY BE LINKED

Sleep apnea involves pauses in breathing or shallow breaths during sleep. The breathing pauses can last from a few seconds to minutes and can occur between five to thirty times or more in an hour. Typically, normal breathing often resumes with a loud snort or choking sound.

During sleep, those with sleep apnea move from deep breathing associated with deep sleep to the shallow breathing of light sleep, with numerous sleep disruptions causing decreased quality of sleep and next-day fatigue.

Millions of American adults have obstructive sleep apnea. Sleep apnea occurs more often in men than in women, and its incidence increases with age. At least one in ten people older than 65 have sleep apnea. Women are more likely to develop sleep apnea during pregnancy and after menopause (because of more belly weight). Sleep apnea is more common in African Americans, Hispanics, and Pacific Islanders. If someone in your family has sleep apnea, you are more likely to develop it.

More than 50 percent of those with sleep apnea are overweight. One cause of sleep apnea is the accumulation of fat deposits in the neck area. These fatty stores press on the tissues of the airway, causing its diameter to narrow. In addition, excess fat stored around the belly presses down on the diaphragm, making breathing strenuous, especially when a person lies on his back during sleep.

Sleep apnea is a stressful disorder because the frequent drops in oxygen level and reduced sleep quality trigger the release of stress hormones that will raise the heart rate and increase the risk of hypertension, heart attack, stroke, irregular heartbeats, obesity, and diabetes. Stress hormones cause blood sugar to rise and insulin to release. As you can see, many of the indications of uncontrolled Met B, prediabetes, and type 2 diabetes are part of sleep apnea: overweight; obesity; hypertension; heart attack; stroke; irregular heartbeat; and more predilections for African Americans, Hispanics, and Pacific Islanders. Most cases of sleep apnea improve when those with uncontrolled Met B, prediabetes, and type 2 diabetes lose weight and control insulin.*

_____

*U.S. Department of Health and Human Services, National Institutes of Health.

provide the quiet, stable internal environment for sleep. When blood sugar drops during the night, you can be abruptly awakened as the brain sends signals for you to eat. Next, your liver releases sugar stores, causing your blood sugar to rise. High blood sugar causes an increased need to urinate, making you feel restless, uncomfortable, and irritable. Peaceful sleep is hard to come by for those with uncontrolled diabetes.

BLURRY VISION AND LIGHT SENSITIVITY (EVEN AT NIGHT)

Certain tissues and organs of the body do *not* require insulin to open the cell's door for blood sugar to enter. The lens of the eye is one of these body parts. A person with normal insulin production always has normal blood sugar and thus has never exposed her eye's lenses to high levels of blood glucose. A person with uncontrolled diabetes regularly absorbs high amounts of sugar directly into the "windshield" of the eye. Excess sugar concentration forces the lens tissue to absorb extra fluid to dilute the excess sugar. For those with uncontrolled diabetes, this excess water content makes their vision appear as if they are looking through a windshield on a rainy day without wipers. Excess fluid causes temporary blurry vision. (If a person with diabetes squints or rubs his eyes, he might notice a momentary clearing of vision because the act of squinting or rubbing physically pushes the excess water out of the lens.) Some people report teary eyes when their blood sugar is high.

At night, lights reflect through the excess fluid pooled in the lenses. Headlights or streetlights seem to be glaringly bright.

Those with uncontrolled blood sugar are more prone to cataracts at an earlier age because their lenses have been accumulating blood sugar over a period of time (like crystallization of the lens). People under the age of 60 who have diabetes are three to four times more likely to develop cataracts.*

---

*H. Cheng, "Causes of Cataract: Age, Sugars and Probably Ultraviolet Radiation," *British Medical Journal* 298 (1989): 1470–1471.

INCREASED ACHES AND PAINS

As with all parts of the human body, nerves and nerve endings are de-signed to reside in an environment of normal blood sugar. When nerve endings are repeatedly exposed to high concentrations of blood sugar, they can become irritated, inflamed, frazzled, or hardened/deadened. Nerves transmit messages from the world to the brain and from the brain to the body. Messages sent back and forth between the brain and our nerves enable us to sense pain, heat, cold, touch, and so on. If the transfer sites on the nerve endings are inflamed or dead-ened, conduction is adversely affected. People with diabetes may ex-perience hypersensation (shooting or burning pain) or constant pain from irritated nerves. Conversely, deadened nerve endings have diffi-culty conducting messages at all, and this failure to communicate can lead to numbness or lack of sensation. (For more on neuropathy, see page 109.)

Whether you have classic symptoms or the quiet bunch of symp-toms that are gradually carrying you toward diabetes, your body is sending you signals that you should not ignore. Knowledge is power, and knowing what is happening in your body is the first step toward making the positive changes that will improve your health and put you in control of your blood glucose.

FINDING OUT: THE DIAGNOSIS

Diabetes is always diagnosed through lab work. You may have had symptoms of diabetes that prompted a blood glucose test, or you may have been symptom-free but as part of an annual physical, your doctor ordered lab work. When the test results were in, depending on the skill, personality, bedside manner, and knowledge of your doctor or health care provider, you may have received your prediabetes or type 2 diabetes diagnosis in one of many ways:

- A personal call from your doctor giving you the "bad news": "I'm sorry to tell you this . . . you have diabetes."
- A message left on your answering machine by the physician's office saying, "You have prediabetes; please watch your sugar and lose weight."
- A terse or disinterested phone call from the office receptionist informing you of your diagnosis. (This call usually comes late in the afternoon on a Friday right before the office closes for the weekend.)
- At your annual physical, a full year after your labs were last drawn and you received no call to inform you that anything was amiss, your doctor reviews your chart and says, "Oh, yes, I see

that you have diabetes . . . you need to lose weight and watch
your sugar intake."

- You had an appointment with your cardiologist who glances at
the lab work forwarded from your general doctor and says, in
passing, "How are you doing with your diabetes?" (You never
knew you had diabetes.)

- You are reading an article in a magazine about the symptoms of
diabetes and realize that you have most of them. At your next
office visit, YOU ask to have diagnostic lab tests and, voilà, you
ARE diabetic.

- Your physician informed you of your diagnosis; recommended
education by a certified diabetes educator; explained the plan of
action; prescribed the correct diet, exercise program, monitoring
schedule, and medications (if necessary); and follows up with
you in eight weeks to check progress.

As a registered dietitian, I've worked one-on-one with people with
Met B, prediabetes, and diabetes for close to thirty years. As a certified
diabetes educator, I've specialized in diabetes management. As a person with type 2 diabetes, I've lived with the disease for fifteen years and
counting.

I know firsthand that when a person gets the phone call or sits
across from a physician and hears the words, "I'm sorry to tell you this,
but you have diabetes," it feels as if the world has suddenly stopped.
Visions of syringes, finger sticks, insulin vials, and dreaded complications spring to mind. Shame quickly follows. *What did I do to myself?
Why didn't I take better care of my body? All that overeating and couch-
potato lifestyle finally caught up to me. I'm a failure. My life will never
be the same. It's all downhill for me.* Some would say that hearing they
had diabetes felt like a life sentence.

Because diabetes has been misunderstood for so many years, it is often presented as a dreaded, hopeless affliction. Many people become

so distraught when they hear the diagnosis of diabetes that they go through a grieving process described by the Kübler-Ross model: five stages of grief that people may experience when dealing with a tragedy. You may have processed the diagnosis of diabetes in one or more of these ways:

Denial. "I feel fine," or "This can't be happening; the test has to be wrong."

Anger. "Why me? It's not fair!" or "I am too young for diabetes," or "Who is to blame?"

Bargaining. "I will do anything . . . just don't let me lose my vision," or "I will never eat cake or ice cream again. Just let the diabetes disappear now."

Depression. "I have diabetes and can't live the way I used to; why bother with anything?" or "I'm going to end up on dialysis like Grandpa . . . what's the point?"

Acceptance. "It's going to be okay," or "I may as well learn to control my sugar."

Accompanying the diagnosis with an apology and condolences is a negative way to present this information to a patient, but this is the way the diagnosis has always been given. Although diabetes can be a serious condition if left untreated, focusing on the negative is an antiquated and incorrect approach. In the twenty-first century, it is no longer valid to present diabetes the same way it was presented in the 1950s, '60s, '70s, '80s, or even the '90s. The information we now know about the disease, its origins, its treatment, and the proper lifestyle that will combat the disease is very different from what we understood just fifteen years ago. It's unfortunate that with all the updated information about diabetes, the way many medical professionals alert patients to the condition is still back in the Stone Ages.

Imagine if you were given the diagnosis in the following manner:

"Mrs. Jones, you have type 2 diabetes. It's a hereditary condition that involves an imbalance of the hormone insulin. It can be controlled with changes in diet and exercise, and perhaps medication. By addressing your diabetes with the proper diet, exercise, and lifestyle, you can live a very happy, healthy life."

Whether you are new to your diagnosis or have had diabetes for years, it's time to really learn about yourself, your body, how you got to this place in your life, and what you can do to live a healthier life than before your diagnosis.

A HORMONAL IMBALANCE, NOT A LIFE SENTENCE

Having diabetes doesn't have to be a life sentence. Unlike a terminal illness, type 2 diabetes is a chronic illness that is always controllable. It is the end result of many years of insulin imbalance in your body. Now that you know you have the diagnosis, you finally know who you really are, and how your particular body works.

If you or someone you know is diagnosed with prediabetes or type 2 diabetes, consider the diagnosis to be a wake-up call: a chance to focus on your physical, emotional, and psychological well-being and become healthier than you were before the diagnosis.

It is actually possible for a person newly diagnosed with type 2 diabetes to walk out the door of the physician's office at the stage of acceptance. "I know I have a medical condition, but thankfully, it is a condition that can be controlled, maybe even without medication. I'm not thrilled to hear the diagnosis, but at least I can do something about it."

From today forward, I'd like to suggest looking at diabetes through a different lens. Instead of viewing the diagnosis as a lightning bolt that struck and left a negative impact on your future, it would be more helpful to think of diabetes as the result of a progressive hormonal imbalance that can be controlled through lifestyle.

If you have controlled Met B, you can prevent prediabetes. If you have prediabetes, you can prevent or greatly delay its progression to type 2 diabetes. If you have diabetes, you can control it on as little medication as possible.

THE LONG AND WINDING ROAD

Although the diagnosis can seem like a shock, your diabetes didn't happen overnight. For those with prediabetes and type 2 diabetes, realize that on the day you were born, you already had the genes that predisposed you to developing blood sugar issues. For years before being diagnosed with type 2 diabetes, you were living with excess insulin production and excess fat deposits on your body and circulating in your blood. You eventually began to develop insulin resistance and then prediabetes. Although you may have a brand-new diagnosis of type 2 diabetes, or your most recent lab work came back with a warning of prediabetes, the way your body processes food and your resultant blood sugar levels have been "just a little off" for a long time. For years before you were diagnosed, your daily blood sugar levels may have been a little lower than average and also a tad higher than normal. You may have started with these small fluctuations, but as the years passed, your blood sugar's levels became roller coaster–like, rising higher and dropping lower—making for a very chaotic ride. During much of this ride, you were most likely unaware that you had boarded the train to type 2 diabetes.

BUT I'M TOO YOUNG TO BE A TYPE 2, "OLD AGE" DIABETIC!

Not many years ago, type 2 diabetes was called adult-onset diabetes and was considered a disease of the elderly. You may recall hearing a grandparent complain that they had a "touch of sugar" or "borderline diabetes," or they had to watch their sugar intake. The diagnosis of type 2 diabetes carried the mental image of someone old, overweight, and barely moving.

Surprisingly, the average age at diagnosis for those with type 2 diabetes is now 46 years.* Because many endocrinologists suggest that a person may have had undiagnosed diabetes for six years before they are actually diagnosed with type 2, the median age of onset is only 40 years of age. Forty is certainly not elderly. In recent years, I've counseled patients as young as 11 years of age with type 2. Type 2 diabetes is now a worldwide epidemic, and the age of onset around the globe is younger than ever. Some believe this is because of improved awareness of symptoms; some believe it is because of tightened criteria for what constitutes diabetes. Others are sure it is because of poor diet, lack of adequate exercise, environmental toxins, or increased stress. Whatever the case, close to 26 million children and adults in the United States have diabetes (diagnosed or undiagnosed), and another 79 million have prediabetes. You are not alone.

Getting Diagnosed: About Your Lab Work

The diagnosis of prediabetes and type 2 diabetes is always made "by the numbers" through your blood work. For proper diagnosis, you should have your fasting blood glucose and hemoglobin A1C levels checked. Most physicians prefer to see two fasting glucose readings or hemoglobin A1C readings out of the normal range on different days before they diagnose diabetes.

Annals of Family Medicine 3, no. 1 (January 2005): 60–63. DOI 10.1370/afm.214.

FASTING BLOOD GLUCOSE

When having a fasting glucose test to rule out diabetes, you should be fasting (water only) for a minimum of eight hours prior to the test or overnight, unless otherwise instructed. You can drink water before your test. It is best to schedule your lab test as early as possible in the morning because every five hours that pass without food, your liver will deposit sugar (from stored glycogen) into your blood. The longer you wait to have your labs drawn, the higher your blood sugar might be. Try to have a snack as late as possible before midnight and have your labs drawn as early as possible the next morning for the most accurate results.

- The better hydrated you are, the easier it is for the lab technician to find a good vein, and the better the blood will flow. When you are under-hydrated, veins collapse and blood volume is decreased.
- Always wash your hands before your lab work and before leaving the lab. I always carry hand sanitizer for use after blood work.
- It's a good idea to bring a snack along. After your blood is drawn, you can immediately eat to get your day started without further delay.

Fasting blood glucose indicates the mg/dL of sugar in your blood at the moment in time when your blood was drawn, after at least eight hours have passed without food.

Fasting Glucose Readings:
- 65–99 mg/dL = normal
- 100–125 mg/dL = elevated, indicating prediabetes
- 126 and higher = diabetes

HEMOGLOBIN A1C

Before the hemoglobin A1C (HbA1C, glycosylated hemoglobin) test was available, patients would be strict with their diet and exercise regimen for a few days prior to their doctor appointment in an effort to create a "better than reality" blood sugar result. The current hemoglobin A1C test shows your average blood sugar for up to ninety days before you go to the lab. How can a test look two to three months backwards in time?

Glucose travels through the blood attached to a protein called hemoglobin. Hemoglobin is present in red blood cells, which have a life span of about three months. In the lab, three-month-old red blood cells' hemoglobin/glucose is measured to show the average blood sugar that was present twenty-four hours a day over the preceding three months. If you had your A1C checked on May 1, it would indicate your average blood sugar for all of February, March, and April.

You do not have to be fasting for a hemoglobin A1C test.

Pregnant women, people who have had recent severe bleeding or blood transfusions, those with chronic kidney or liver disease, or those with iron or vitamin B12 anemia *should not* use HbA1C to diagnose diabetes because these conditions can skew the results.

HbA1C Readings:
- 5.0–5.6 percent = (32–38mmol/mol) = normal
- 5.7–6.4 percent (39–46 mmol/mol) = prediabetes
- 6.5 percent (47 mmol/mol) and higher = diabetes

Although the ADA recommends that people with type 2 diabetes maintain HbA1C under 7.0 percent, the stricter American Association of Clinical Endocrinologists recommends HbA1C at less than 6.5 percent.

HbA1C is an average of highs and lows in blood sugar that occur over a two- to three-month period of time. A person with normal blood sugar who does not experience wide fluctuations in blood sugar can

Assessing Elevated Blood Sugar

According to the 2007 guidelines issued by the American Association of Clinical Endocrinologists, the following levels are diagnostic of blood sugar issues:

Prediabetes:
- fasting blood sugar of 100–125 mg/dL (5.56–6.94 mmol/L)
- blood sugar of 140–199 mg/dL (7.78–11.06 mmol/L) two hours after ingesting 75 grams of glucose

Diabetes:
- fasting blood sugar of 126 mg/dL (7 mmol/L) or greater
- random ("casual") blood sugar of 200 mg/dL (11.11 mmol/L) or greater, plus symptoms of diabetes

If there's any doubt about the diagnosis, testing should be repeated on a subsequent day.

FASTING BLOOD GLUCOSE and HbA1C

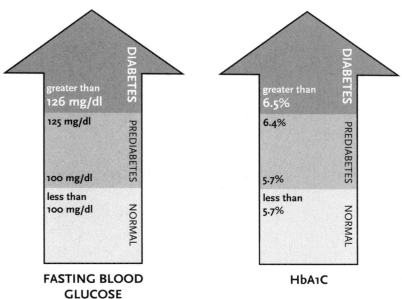

have an A1C of 5.5. A person taking medication to control diabetes can achieve the same average blood sugar, but it may be the result of the average of very high and very low readings that ultimately average out to a normal A1C. For people who take medication to lower blood glucose, I never look at an A1C as a be all/end all. I always look at their A1C in the context of daily home blood sugar monitoring results.

KEEPING TRACK OF YOUR LAB WORK

Have you ever noticed that when the results of your lab work are back, getting a copy of the results can be challenging? I recommend that when you are at the office, you ask your physician for a copy, or you can ask the nurse or doctor who calls your home to discuss your results to forward a copy. You might also consider asking your doctor's office to scan and email your results or provide your doctor's office with a stamped, self-addressed envelope and a request for a copy of your lab results. Keep your lab results in a file so that you can compare tests from year to year. You might even use a chart (see page 340 for an example) to track the progress of your blood tests.

The diagnosis tells you what you have, but it is important to understand the genetic and lifestyle factors that lead to your diagnosis.

UNDERSTANDING METABOLISM

Long ago, I came to realize that the human body is the most intricate, sophisticated, and perfectly designed machine. The body has backup systems that have backup systems, with the sole purpose to keep this ultimate machine alive and running—living, if you will.

Think of your body like an automobile. To keep the car running in tip-top shape, you must take care of and maintain it. There must be proper fueling (healthy diet, fluid intake, vitamins and minerals) with the right octane gas (healthy blood sugar). The car cannot remain parked in a garage forever; it must be taken out for a regular spin (exercise) and have regularly scheduled maintenance and tune-ups (medical checkups and minor procedures as needed) to make sure all the parts are working properly.

You would never invest in a car and then refuse to put the proper octane gas in its tank, ignore its fluid levels, let it sit in a garage undriven, ignore scheduled maintenance, or fail to get a tune-up. If you did, your car would work less efficiently, and after a period of time, it would break. Eventually, such neglect would result in the car failing to run.

The body also requires proper fuel, adequate activity, rest periods, and scheduled maintenance. A neglected body runs less and less efficiently. Sometimes the process of body-part fatigue is slow, and the body's owner is oblivious to its downward spiral, gradually becoming tolerant of (and accustomed to) its aches, pains, and irregularities. After a period of time, without necessary care or repair, the body eventually breaks down with illness or major damage.

Healthy babies are born into the world with a top-of-the-line machine, the equivalent of a Ferrari. Unfortunately, most of us live our lives not really understanding how this machine functions. (We don't even get a basic owner's manual.) Perhaps if we truly understood the gift we have and how to care for it properly, we could maintain better health for the long term.

I find that people tend to take their bodies for granted until something goes wrong. We might not pay attention to what we eat; we might skimp on sleep; we might drink a little too much alcohol or become couch potatoes until our physician tells us some dire health news, such as, "You have four blocked arteries and need bypass surgery." "You had a mild heart attack." "Your liver enzymes are elevated." "You have lung cancer." It sometimes takes a kick in the pants or a brush with death to get a person motivated to take the proper care of himself. Because diabetes is a progressive disease, there are warning signs that, if heeded, can put you back in the driver's seat to take control of your health and well-being.

My ultimate goal has always been to get to the root of medical problems at the base level and to ascertain if diet, exercise, lifestyle changes, and so on can remedy the problem in a natural way. I'm fairly certain that the majority of health problems are caused by or exacerbated by people who knowingly or unknowingly damaged their machine. I am also sure that the human body was not meant to require chemicals to temporarily fix problems.

From the perspective of taking proper care of yourself, I think it helps to know how a machine works from the inside out. To study a body system, it helps to break it down to its base parts, to learn how these parts are meant to work on their own, and then come to understand how they link to other body parts to work in an integrated system. When you understand the parts and how they should relate, you can finally make sense of what happens when a part breaks down and what backup systems come into play.

Call it serendipity, call it chance, but the organ system that always fascinated me the most was the endocrine system. At the time I "fell hard" for the endocrine system, I had no idea that it was the organ system that was already breaking down in my own body.

The endocrine system is involved with almost every cell, organ, and function of your body. It is made up of glands and hormones: A gland is a group of cells that produce and release hormones, chemical messengers that transfer information from one set of cells to another. Glands release the hormones directly into the blood, and they travel to a certain location to pass along their chemical message. Hormones connect to receptors on specific target cells. An example is the hormone insulin, which is released by the pancreas and travels to fat and muscle cells, attaches to insulin receptors, and enables glucose from the blood to feed the cells. The cells need glucose like a car's engine needs gas.

More than thirty hormones regulate your bodily functions, including your heart beat, the speed of your metabolism, the breakdown and processing of food, your response to stress, the onset of puberty, the onset and duration of menopause, fertility, body temperature, and sleep cycle. There are so many body systems influenced by the endocrine system, yet this system is rarely discussed or understood.

THE THYROID GLAND

Hormones produced by the thyroid gland determine the speed at which your body functions; your metabolic rate. A slow metabolism can lead to weight gain or the inability to lose weight, but only 6–8 percent of the population has hypothyroidism. Because of a hormonal imbalance involving thyroid stimulating hormone (TSH), hypothyroidism causes a slower than normal metabolic rate.

There is no guesswork involved in determining if you have hypothyroidism; a simple blood test including a thyroid panel will show if your thyroid is working properly. If diagnosed with hypothyroidism, your physician will prescribe a hormone supplement for you in the dose needed to bring your TSH into the normal range.

Almost every patient I see for weight reduction tells me that at some point in her life she was sure she had a slow metabolism. Her physician tested her thyroid (via a blood test) and found that the thyroid was functioning normally. Most of these patients say they were disheartened to hear that their thyroid function was normal because now they had no explanation as to why they could not lose weight despite a healthy diet and exercise.

WHAT IS METABOLISM?

Metabolism is a word that is loosely tossed around in the media these days. "Tips to increase metabolism," "Foods that speed up your metabolism," and "How to jumpstart your slow metabolism" are headlines for magazine articles and hot topics for talk shows largely because it is believed that a great number of people have slow metabolic rates, which are hampering their weight-loss attempts.

In a nutshell, metabolism consists of the sum total of all the body processes necessary to maintain life. Heartbeat, respiration, digestion, kidney function, and even brain function are all part of metabolism. The number of calories it takes to run the body (not including the calories needed for physical activity) can be determined by the Harris-Benedict equation for base metabolic rate (BMR) or basal energy expenditure (BEE). The formula takes into account a person's gender, age, height, and current weight. It does not take into account calories needed for physical activity or movement.

WOMEN:

BMR calculation for women using kg   BMR = 655.1 + (9.563 x weight in kg) + (1.850 x height in cm) – (4.676 x age in years)

BMR calculation for women using pounds   BMR = 655 + (4.35 x weight in pounds) + (4.7 x height in inches) – (4.7 x age in years)

MEN:

BMR calculation for men using kg   BMR = 66.5 + (13.75 x weight in kg) + (5.003 x height in cm) – (6.775 x age in years)

BMR calculation for men using pounds   BMR = 66 + (6.23 x weight in pounds) + (12.7 x height in inches) – (6.76 x age in years)

RAISING YOUR METABOLIC RATE

You can see that the only factor in the Harris-Benedict equation that you can possibly manipulate is your weight because you are locked into your gender, age, and height. Ironically, the more you weigh, the higher your metabolic calorie burn is. It should be obvious that no food, drink, chili pepper, or trick can influence this equation. It is what it is.

If you want to increase the calories you burn in a day and to increase your metabolic rate, there are only two things you can do—one is healthy, the other is not:

1. Healthy approach: increase physical activity (develops metabolically active muscle tissue and stimulates heart rate and bodily functions);
2. Unhealthy approach: chemically manipulate heart rate (artificially and temporarily stimulates heart rate with no change in muscle tissue).

In addition to the calories deduced from the Harris-Benedict equation, another factor that determines caloric requirement is physical activity. The more you exercise in terms of regularity, duration, and intensity, the more calories you will burn. The more exercise you do, the more metabolically active muscle tissue you develop. More muscle tissue means more calories burned all day, every day.

Let's see how this plays out with three women who are the same age, height, and weight but who have differing activity levels. Each woman is 28 years old, 5 feet 5 inches, and 136 pounds, and all have a BMR of 1,421. One woman is an athlete in training, one is moderately active, and one is sedentary.

Little to no exercise   Daily calories needed = BMR x 1.2

Light exercise
(1–3 days per week)   Daily calories needed = BMR x 1.375

Moderate exercise
(3–5 days per week)   Daily calories needed = BMR x 1.55

Heavy exercise
(6–7 days per week)   Daily calories needed = BMR x 1.725

Very heavy exercise
(twice per day, extra
heavy workouts)   Daily calories needed = BMR x 1.9

Very active woman: multiply BMR by 1.725 —
BMR= 1421 x 1.725 = 2451 calories/day to maintain 136 pounds

Moderately active woman: multiply BMR by 1.55 —
BMR= 1421 x 1.55 = 2202 calories/day to maintain 136 pounds

Sedentary woman: multiply BMR by 1.2 —
BMR = 1421 x 1.2 = 1705 calories/day to maintain 136 pounds

The very active, athletic woman can consume 746 more calories per day than the sedentary woman to maintain the same weight.

You can easily see how by simply becoming active, people of the same gender, age, height, and weight can burn more calories per day and actually change the body's composition to replace fat tissue with active muscle tissue. More muscle tissue will burn more calories throughout the day.

DIET PILLS AND OTHER ARTIFICIAL STIMULANTS

Another way to raise metabolic rate is to artificially manipulate your heart rate, respiratory rate, and speed of other organ systems by taking diet pills or other stimulants. Stimulants force the heart to beat quicker and the lungs to breathe faster The downside to using stimulants is that the increase in heart rate is artificial and temporary. When you no longer take the stimulant, your heart rate and body speed immediately return to normal.

Taking diet pills or stimulants is like running a marathon without a finish line—your body is going and going without stopping. The artificial stimulants keep your heart overpumping for hours, tiring the heart muscle without giving it a chance to rest. Your heart races, your breathing quickens, your thoughts race—you are literally on speed.

Another major concern is that when you stop taking the artificial stimulants, your heart rate, respiration, thinking, and all other bodily functions will immediately return to normal. To you, this feels like a crash, and you will want to take the products again. Being stuck in this cycle means you are now addicted to speed. Aside from the wear and tear this puts on your body, you will not achieve the weight-loss results you desire. In fact, when you stop taking the pills, every single ounce of weight you lost through artificial manipulation will return almost overnight. Because you didn't develop any new muscle, you have not increased your metabolic furnaces. Revving up your metabolism through artificial means is a terrible plan. Don't ever try it . . . it never, ever works.

DANGER!

Many people with Met B, prediabetes, and type 2 diabetes have multiple metabolic medical conditions other than their weight, such as hypertension, partially blocked or hardened blood vessels, elevated lipids (fats), and inflamed nerve endings. Adding diet pills and artificial stimulants to this situation can be deadly.

METABOLISM A VERSUS METABOLISM B: IT'S IN YOUR GENES

There appear to be genetic differences that determine the way a body processes food. In the case of Metabolism A versus Metabolism B, we are looking specifically at the processing of the energy nutrient, carbohydrate.

Metabolism A, or "textbook" metabolism, is the metabolism explained in medical books and presumed to be prevalent in most people. It operates in hormonal equilibrium. An alternate metabolism, which I call Metabolism B, is the underlying metabolic state for millions of people. Those with uncontrolled Met B gain weight around the middle and experience progressively increasing blood pressure, glucose, LDL cholesterol, depression, anxiety, and fatigue.

Although you are born with the genetic propensity for Met B, it appears that environmental triggers (stress, overweight, inactivity, illness, and certain medications) trigger the onset of symptoms that begin quietly and eventually overtake your physical, emotional, and psychological quality of life.

According to the ADA, if one of your parents developed type 2 diabetes after age 50, the chances of your developing diabetes is 1 in 13. If your parent's diagnosis came before age 50, your chances increase to 1 in 7. If both your mom and dad have type 2 diabetes, your risk increases to a 1 in 2 chance.

Besides the genetic link, life stressors (including excess weight, physical inactivity, emotional stress, illness, perhaps food additives or toxins) seem to progressively push the metabolic changes that eventually result in type 2 diabetes.

If you currently have prediabetes or type 2 diabetes, you were most likely born with a genetic predisposition for Metabolism B. Most people mistakenly believe that anyone who gains excess fat is eating too many calories, overconsuming sugar and sweets, living on fast food, and being inactive. They also believe that anyone can eat their way into type 2 diabetes—that anyone who lives the lifestyle I just described WILL develop diabetes in time.

After working in the field of medical nutrition for more than thirty years, I can tell you that some very overweight people do not have nor will they ever develop diabetes. There appears to be a genetic component that must be engaged for type 2 diabetes to occur.

METABOLISM A, METABOLISM B, AND THE PRETZEL BOMB

Food contains three macronutrients: carbohydrate, protein, and fat. Of these three nutrients, the body's preferred source of energy is carbohydrate (50 to 60 percent of protein and 10 percent of fat can turn to blood sugar, but the process is much slower and less efficient).

Examples of carbohydrate foods (the primary energy source for the human body): milk, fruit, breads, rice, pasta, legumes, sweets, grains, chips, pretzels, crackers, cookies, ice cream. To understand the quirky metabolism that can eventually result in diabetes, you should first understand the normal metabolism of someone with Met A.

When two people with differing metabolisms eat the same thing, in this case a soft pretzel, their bodies react quite differently to the carbohydrate.

Metabolism A. This person eats the soft pretzel, and 100 percent of its net carbohydrate grams convert to blood sugar. As blood sugar rises, the pancreas releases the correct amount of insulin. Insulin enters the bloodstream in search of muscle and fat cells with insulin receptors.

If the person has not exercised and muscle cells are not currently asking to be refilled with blood sugar stores, the majority of insulin keys will connect to fat cells. The insulin key opens the fat cell by fitting the insulin receptor like a key fits a lock. The correct amount of insulin opens the right number of cells (muscle or fat), enabling blood sugar to leave the bloodstream and fill the opened cells. When the process is complete, the sugar remaining in the bloodstream is always in the normal range. Equilibrium = normalcy = all's well.

Metabolism B. The Met B person eats the pretzel, and 100 percent of its net carbohydrate grams convert to blood sugar. As blood sugar rises, the pancreas releases just a little extra insulin (perhaps due to a genetic tendency). If the person has not exercised, and muscle cells are not requesting to be refilled with blood sugar, the majority of insulin will move to fat cells. The insulin keys will connect to the fat cell doors by fitting the insulin receptors.

What happens next is the defining moment in how Met B operates differently in reaction to carbohydrate. If you come to understand what follows, you will see exactly why those with Met B gain weight around the middle and end up with increased blood pressure, glucose, LDL cholesterol, triglycerides, depression, anxiety, and fatigue. The extra insulin keys will connect and open excess fat cells that now require to be fed blood sugar. The bloodstream will accommodate and fill these excess fat cells with sugar, leaving the sugar remaining in the bloodstream a little lower than normal.

This low blood sugar level is sensed by the brain. The Met B person's brain gives a signal to "eat more carbohydrate now, your blood sugar is too low." The Met B person begins to feel a little hungry, a little

THE PRETZEL BOMB

Depending upon your metabolism, a pretzel can cause two very different reactions in the body. This chart illustrates how the paths diverge.

You and your friend both eat a pretzel.

The pretzel's carbohydrate turns to blood glucose and enters the bloodstream.

The brain senses the blood glucose rise and instructs
the pancreas to release the hormone insulin.

METABOLISM A
AND THE PRETZEL

The pancreas releases exactly
the right amount of insulin to handle
the rise in blood glucose.

Insulin acts like a key and opens the right
amount of fat and muscle cells and returns the
glucose in the bloodstream to normal.

Glucose from the pretzel provides immediate
energy, replaces glycogen in muscle and liver,
and any excess is stored as fat.

Equilibrium results in the body feeling
satisfied and full after the meal.

Satisfaction lasts for four to five hours
until hunger naturally occurs..

METABOLISM B (YOU)
AND THE PRETZEL

The pancreas overreacts and releases excess
insulin to handle the rise in blood glucose.

Excess insulin opens excess fat cells,
ushers in the glucose and leaves too little
glucose in the blood for basic energy.
Your fat cells get microscopically larger
and receptors "stretch" a bit.

The brain signals you to eat more carbohydrate
to quickly raise the blood glucose.
You feel hungry, tired, shaky, nauseated,
and irritable until you eat a carbohydrate snack.

You temporarily feel better
as blood glucose rises.

Your brain senses a rise in blood glucose and
tells the pancreas to once again release insulin.

Your pancreas overreleases again
and the cycle repeats itself.

empty, with a slight craving for another bite of a pretzel or a piece of chocolate or maybe a scoop of ice cream. (These foods, all carbohydrates, will then boost the lagging blood sugar.)

If the person with Met B chooses to eat, the carbohydrate in the snack will cause the blood sugar to rise again, and the pancreas will release just a little too much insulin again—and the vicious cycle replays. Slowly but surely, the person with Met B is getting fatter; the fat cells themselves are growing in size and stretching. The insulin receptors that are meant to fit the person's insulin perfectly will slowly begin to change shape. Little by little, the fat cells grow in size, and insulin receptors become misshapen. This is what is known as "insulin resistance."

Now, what if the Met B person did not answer the craving to eat that extra carbohydrate food? What if she ignored the brain's cues to eat carbs to help boost the lagging blood sugar? Would this break the cycle and enable the person to lose weight and develop normally shaped insulin receptors?

Unfortunately, the answer is NO. The human body is a complex machine with built-in survival mechanisms. If she didn't heed the brain's prodding her to snack and raise that bloodsugar, the brain would shift gears to Plan B.

Plan B. The brain requires the correct level of blood sugar to function normally. If blood sugar drops and the person doesn't refill the tank by eating more carbohydrate, the brain sends a hormonal signal to another organ: the liver. One of the liver's many functions is to release stored blood sugar (glycogen) into the bloodstream at the request of the brain.

So, the liver would release glycogen, and blood sugar would rise whether she snacked or not. The rise in blood sugar would trigger the pancreas to release insulin. The Met B pancreas would release just a little too much insulin, excess fat cells would be opened, and excess sugar would be removed from the bloodstream and stored as fat. Over time, this person would slowly get fatter from feeding excess fat cells, the fat cells would slowly grow, and the connection between the insulin receptor and insulin would lessen. At this early stage in the progression of Met B to diabetes, the person's average blood sugar (HbA1C) could be normal or even lower than normal. When I see an A1C under 5.3, I'm thinking, this might be the very beginning of the symptoms of Met B.

GAINING WEIGHT WHILE YOU SLEEP?

A person with the genetic predisposition to Met B is not even safe when she's asleep. In normal physiology, the liver releases sugar stores whenever a person fails to eat carbohydrate (energy) foods on a regular basis. Besides providing an emergency lift if blood sugar dips lower than normal, the liver also self-feeds when we take too long between meals, when we skip meals, and even when we sleep. This self-feeding mechanism of the liver is not unique to people with Met B. The human liver is on a five-hour clock—that is, whenever a person goes beyond five hours without eating, the liver receives a hormonal signal to release sugar stores. This is not a "when I'm awake" clock. The body's five-hour clock is operational twenty-four hours a day.

Every night when we sleep, there will be gaps of more than five hours without eating carbohydrate. When the fifth hour passes, the liver will automatically release blood sugar. In the body of someone with normal metabolism, the correct amount of insulin will be released to accommodate this rise in blood sugar. When the person with Met B's pancreas overreleases insulin, the same fat-building chain of events that happens during the day also occurs during the night.

PHIL AND LISA

Phil has a weight problem. He has been listening to TV talk shows that proclaim, "If you want to lose weight, don't eat after 7 PM." But Phil unknowingly has Met B. If he does not eat after 7 PM, his liver will automatically self-feed every five hours until he eats the next day. This is an automatic process similar to the kidneys filtering, the brain processing information, the lungs breathing, and the heart beating. It happens without the person's consciously taking any action to trigger these body functions.

This liver release of sugar occurs approximately every five hours during the day if a person skips a meal or snack and also during sleep whether you have Met A or Met B. The difference is how the person's pancreas responds to the liver's normal around-the-clock feeding help:

Lisa (Metabolism A)

6:00 PM—Lisa has dinner, doesn't snack afterward, and goes to bed at 10:00 PM.

11:00 PM—Lisa's liver releases glycogen, and her pancreas responds with a normal amount of insulin that opens the appropriate number of cells. Her blood sugar is stable for 4–5 hours. Sleep is restful and sound, with smooth blood sugar fueling the body's functions.

4:00 AM—liver releases glycogen and blood sugar remains normal.

9:00 AM—same. Because Lisa did not eat yet, her liver will release glycogen, and blood sugar will be regulated.

9:15 AM—Lisa has breakfast.

Phil (Uncontrolled Metabolism B)

6:00 PM—Phil joins Lisa for dinner, doesn't snack afterward, and goes to bed at 10:00 PM.

11:00 PM to 9:15 AM: Phil's liver releases glycogen beginning at approximately 11:00 PM every few hours until approximately 9:00 AM, and his pancreas responds with excess insulin that opens excess fat cells, leaving his blood sugar lower than normal. Because he is in bed for the night, he doesn't eat anything to bring the blood sugar back up. His liver again releases glycogen to normalize low blood sugar; excess insulin is again released. Excess fat cells receive sugar, and blood sugar dips again. The liver again releases glycogen to normalize the sugar, and the cycle continues until Phil awakens (tired from his roller-coaster blood sugar ride) and eats his first meal. During the night, his liver has self-fed, and over and over his pancreas responded with excess insulin. He awakens microscopically fatter than Lisa without having eaten more calorically.

In Phil's case, and the case of anyone with uncontrolled Met B, as time passes, his pancreas gradually tires from the excess insulin release that occurs around the clock. As the pancreas fatigues, it makes less and less insulin. After years of being overfed, fat cells have grown (Phil is now overweight and has a roll of fat around his middle), and his insulin receptors have become misshapen. He has prediabetes that, if uncontrolled, will ultimately progress to full-blown, irreversible type 2 diabetes.

DETERMINING IF YOU HAVE MET A OR MET B

There are subclinical symptoms that someone with uncontrolled Met B feels on a daily basis: fatigue, mild depression, carb binges, brain fog, inability to focus and concentrate, midline fat, easy weight gain and difficult weight loss, restless sleep, decreased libido, and blurry vision. It also is possible to have an objective marker of the beginning of uncontrolled Met B in a person's blood work years before they are diagnosed with prediabetes and many years before they would become type 2 diabetic.

WHAT YOU CAN DO—REQUEST THE TESTS

In my private practice, I specialize in weight reduction and diabetes management. For more than fifteen years, I have required that my patients bring fasting lab work to their initial weight loss session, as I cannot help a person to choose the best weight loss program unless I know the type of metabolism they have.

I recommend that you ask your physician to test the following blood markers. They should be retested at least annually to keep tabs on what is happening inside of your body. Make sure that you are fasting (no food at least eight hours before blood is drawn).

Fasting glucose (sugar in your blood after eight hours of not eating) can be measured as follows:
- Normal: most labs use 65–99 mg/dL as normal
- Uncontrolled Met B reference range: less than 70 mg/dL or greater than or equal to 89 mg/dL
- Prediabetes: 100–125 mg/dL
- Diabetes: greater than or equal to 126 mg/dL

Total cholesterol (the sum total of LDL, HDL and other fats in your blood) may be as follows:
- Normal: less than 200 mg/dL
- Uncontrolled Met B reference range: greater than 200 mg/dL

LDL cholesterol (low density lipoprotein, also known as bad cholesterol) measures as follows:
- Normal: less than 130 mg/dL
- Uncontrolled Met B reference range: greater than 99 mg/dL

HDL cholesterol (high density lipoprotein, also known as good cho-
lesterol) measures as follows:
- Normal reference range: greater than 45 mg/dL
- Uncontrolled Met B reference range: less than 45 mg/dL

Triglycerides (a form of fat in the blood and fat tissue) is as follows:
- Normal reference range: less than 150 mg/dL
- Uncontrolled Met B reference range: less than 50 mg/dL
  or greater than or equal to 100 mg/dL

TSH (thyroid stimulating hormone) measures thus:
- Normal reference range: 0.45–4.5*

Hemoglobin (Hb) A1C (measures the amount of blood sugar car-
ried by red blood cells over the past three months, thus providing an
indication of your average blood sugar for those months) is as follows:
- Normal: 5.0–5.6 percent
- Uncontrolled Met B reference range: less than 5.3 percent;
  greater than 5.6 percent
- Prediabetes: 5.7–6.4 percent
- Diabetes: greater than or equal to 6.5 percent

Vitamin D, which measures the amount of the storage form of Vita-
min D, 25(OH) D present in your blood, appears this way:
- Normal reference range: greater than 32
- Uncontrolled Met B reference range: less than 40

---

*In 2009, the American Academy of Clinical Endocrinologists (AACE) narrowed the
normal reference range of TSH to 0.3–3.0. This move doubled the number of people
with TSH out of normal range who would now be classified as having hypothyroidism.
Check with your doctor or lab to determine what reference range is considered normal.

"NORMAL" TEST RESULTS

Within minutes of analyzing fasting lab work, I can easily ascertain if the patient has Met A or Met B. (Remember, patients who are at the beginning of symptoms of Met B are not yet sick, and their labs may show readings still considered in the normal range regarding lipid panel or glucose.) My goal is to ascertain where they are on the spectrum of normal target ranges. If I have prior test results, it's really effective to show the patient the progression of certain lab values as time passes. Uncontrolled Met B leaves a progressive path, with steady and gradual changes in several labs. Labs that are a year apart can show significant change, although both sets of labs are still within the normal target range.

With the time constraints placed on physicians these days because of insurance reimbursement, I've noticed that many physicians don't follow the trending in labs. They look at the lab work in front of them rather than looking in spreadsheet fashion to see if there are changes occurring over time.

If a patient came to me with the following normal lab work (their labs are all within typical reference ranges on lab reports), I can point out the beginning of uncontrolled Metabolism B.

- Fasting glucose of 91   (Uncontrolled Met B = results greater than or equal to 89)
- Hb A1C of 5.1   (Uncontrolled Met B = results less than 5.3)
- Triglycerides of 103   (Uncontrolled Met B = results greater than or equal to 100)
- LDL of 108   (Uncontrolled Met B = results greater than 99)
- Vitamin D of 36   (Uncontrolled Met B = results under 40)

Most of these labs would not be flagged on a lab slip as being out of target range. Yet all these labs can occur as the result of excess insulin. Over time and left untreated, this person's glucose, A1C, LDL cholesterol, triglycerides, and fasting insulin will rise, and Vitamin D levels will fall into the danger zone. This progression might take months, it might take years, but left untreated . . . it will happen.

If I see a patient who is beginning to show the lab results of someone with uncontrolled Met B, I am practically certain that she has been told that her labs are normal, and some patients have even been congratulated on having good lab work.

Remember that labs are flagged high or low when they fall into a diagnosable unhealthy range perceived as indicating that there might be a medical problem to treat. I prefer to take a proactive look at lab work and study trending in a patient's lab work, which allows a look inside the body for signs of things to come. This is a positive way to look at labs instead of looking at them from the band-aid perspective.

My overview of lab work is often very different from a physician's perspective. The physician is looking for red flags—diagnoses that can be made through lab test results that fall out of the reference normal range. I prefer to look at the whole picture, and in the case of the train ride to diabetes, it is possible to see into the future once certain labs begin to shift.

Remember that a person should be advised of prediabetes when fasting blood glucose is 100–125 mg/dL or HbA1C is 5.7–6.4 mg/dL. Some patients never hear the news that they are in the red zone of prediabetes and know nothing of their blood sugar problems until they are solidly in the diabetes range, with fasting blood glucose more than 125 mg/dL. They are at the point of no return and will always have diabetes.

Long before a diagnosis of prediabetes, changes can be seen in fasting lab work. For years, I have been alerting my patients to their Met

B, and I base their diet program on this delineation. A proactive approach can spare them from becoming prediabetic or developing type 2 diabetes.

My patient would know in advance that although his lab work is currently considered normal by the medical establishment, it shows a trend in his body most likely due to excess insulin release.

Lower numbers are not always better. Lower often indicates the beginning of the train ride.

As previously mentioned, standard labs provide a normal reference range and different laboratories may set slightly different reference ranges. As you look at your lab work, any readings that fall outside of the normal reference range will be flagged with an L (if they are lower than the norm) or H (if they are higher than the norm).

Over the years, I've noticed that when a lab value is marked with an H, the patient is usually alerted. However, lab values that are marked L often go unnoticed, unmentioned, and in some cases are considered to be superior readings.

For example, an HbA1C of 4.8 may be marked L, but many patients are told they have an excellent low A1C. A low HbA1C would mean that the patient has had a low average blood sugar for the previous three months. The same misconception might happen with a low fasting blood glucose result on the lab slip. A fasting glucose of 63 will be flagged L, but the doctor may never focus on it, surmising that lower is better.

The truth is that a fasting glucose of 63 and an A1C of 4.8 can both be indicators of excess insulin release and the beginning of Met B. These low readings (products of excess insulin release and perhaps an overworking pancreas) can give the patient a heads-up that he is a potential candidate for type 2 diabetes in the future. Following the Diabetes Miracle lifestyle can change his future health and medical history. In short, it can change his life.

So, let's assume that the doctor does not mention that low fasting glucose and lower than normal A1C are indicators of Met B. She advises her patient to lose weight based on a traditional low-calorie, low-fat, and low-cholesterol diet. As time passes, his lab work will begin to show the gradual fatiguing of the pancreas and resistance to insulin when his fasting glucose eventually crosses over the 99 mg/dL mark. At this time, hemoglobin A1C is now 5.7. It's time to tell the patient that he has prediabetes and advise him to follow the traditional diet with an added restriction of sugar.

In time and left untreated, this gentleman (who now has inadvertently advanced his pancreas's fatigue to prediabetes) will most likely advance to irreversible type 2 diabetes. With type 2 diabetes, fasting blood sugar exceeds 125 mg/dL, and hemoglobin A1C is 6.5 percent or more.

After years of excess insulin production, the body's fat cells get larger, and insulin does not fit properly (insulin resistance), which in turn leads to pancreas fatigue and the progression from Metabolism B to prediabetes, and ultimately to type 2 diabetes.

And so, because of uncontrolled Met B, the years before a person develops prediabetes or type 2 diabetes are years of excess fat storage, both on the body and in the bloodstream, resulting in belly fat, love handles, muffin top, and back fat as well as increased LDL cholesterol and triglycerides. The train to diabetes lumbers down the tracks. . . .

THE CONNECTION BETWEEN METABOLISM B, OVERWEIGHT, AND DIABETES

A myth exists that all people with excess fat overeat calorically and don't get adequate physical activity. The myth goes on to purport that those with unhealthy eating habits and lack of exercise will necessarily develop type 2 diabetes. As a medical nutritional specialist, I am here to tell you that these myths are false. Type 2 diabetes has a genetic component.

Genes + environmental triggers = uncontrolled Met B
$\xrightarrow{\text{leads to}}$ prediabetes $\xrightarrow{\text{leads to}}$ type 2 diabetes.

Your genes are responsible for such characteristics as a cleft in your chin, the color of your eyes, or the shape of your nose. Mutations in genes can be responsible, in part, for medical conditions we develop over the course of our lifetimes. When you read that "diabetes is inherited," the real truth most likely involves inheriting the predisposition to develop type 2 diabetes, in addition to exposure to environmental factors. Diabetes most likely involves mutations in multiple genes; this is why finding a cure is not as simple as finding "the diabetes gene."

Disorders that seem to be caused by a combination of environmental factors and mutations in multiple genes are known as multifactorial inheritance disorders. Heart disease, hypertension, diabetes, arthritis, cancer, obesity, and Alzheimer's disease are all considered to be multifactorial disorders, the result of multiple genes and multiple environmental factors. One of the factors that contributes to diabetes is how carbohydrates are metabolized.

THE LAW OF CALORIES

It appears that the way your body metabolizes food may involve multiple genes and multiple environmental factors. For years, it was assumed that everyone's metabolism worked in the same way to process nutrients and that body weight was determined by the "universal law of calories": your weight is equal to the total calories you consume minus the total calories you burn.

This "calories in, calories out" philosophy meant that if you desired to lose weight, all you needed to do was to consume fewer calories and pump up your activity—a simple formula. As a result, almost all weight loss diets through the ages have been based on this law of calories. Whether a person is counting points, having diet food delivered to their home, exchanging foods between lists, or using calorie-counting books, he is following a program based on the law of calories. Those with textbook metabolism (Met A) can succeed with calorie-based diets. They can succeed in losing weight by counting points and using diet food deliveries, calorie-based diets, or freeze-dried diet foods.

But at some point in their lives, more than half the people who struggle with weight come to the realization that traditional diets no longer work for them. They might find themselves thinking: "How much less can I eat and how much more can I exercise? My friends all eat more than I do and exercise less, and they are all so much thinner." From my research and other research on metabolic syndrome, prediabetes, and type 2 diabetes, more than 50 percent of people who struggle with weight loss cannot succeed by following this universal law of calories. As we have seen in the previous chapter, the root cause of the inability to lose weight using conventional diets is uncontrolled Met B.

METABOLISM AND DIABETES

In the 1950s, medical researchers began to discuss a compilation of medical conditions that would become known as metabolic syndrome (or Syndrome X). The medical conditions have since been linked together in a package that includes midline fat deposits, elevated total cholesterol, low HDL cholesterol, high LDL cholesterol, elevated triglycerides, elevated blood pressure, and elevated blood sugar. These conditions were called a syndrome because they often appeared in a cluster. The conditions do not begin at the same time, and they are progressive in nature. As time passes, the medical conditions progressively become worse and in time will require medication.

With a limited knowledge of what linked these conditions, it was very clear that left untreated, these medical aberrations could absolutely lead to heart disease (heart attack), vascular disease (stroke), diabetic complications, obesity, and more. Because the conditions appeared to be fat-related—midline fat deposits (belly fat or apple shape), cholesterol, triglycerides, blood pressure—speculation centered around the need to lower the total fat grams, cholesterol grams, calories, sugar content, and sodium in the diet of those with metabolic syndrome.

Because of this mind-set, people with Metabolism B, prediabetes, and type 2 diabetes have always been prescribed a diet similar to the 1400-calorie ADA, low-fat, low-cholesterol, and low-sodium diet. It is a difficult lifestyle to follow as there are so many restrictions. But more frustrating than living the lifestyle was the fact that it never halted metabolic syndrome nor its progression to overweight or type 2 diabetes.

To this day, dietitians and physicians all over the United States and world are recommending the above diet restrictions. Despite adhering to all the restrictions, people with Met B, prediabetes, or type 2 diabetes do not succeed on this traditional diet, and their metabolic syndrome worsens. More and more medications are added, and doses are increased in an attempt to medicinally normalize the progressive medical maladies.

The reason this strict diet fails to work is not the fault of the dieter. The problem is that this diet approach never matched the root cause: the hormonal imbalance of the fat-gain hormone insulin. Decreasing calories, dietary cholesterol, fat grams, simple sugar, and sodium does not address insulin release. It is not the dieter's fault that she didn't lose weight or get healthier. The diet never halted the progression of metabolic syndrome and in fact seems to have made the syndrome worse and with faster progression.

Despite the fact that the diet and exercise program we've recommended for years does not work for the millions suffering from metabolic syndrome, it is prescribed to this day—a day in which diabetes and obesity have evolved into epidemics.

How Does Uncontrolled Metabolism B Ultimately Lead to Type 2 Diabetes?

When I began focusing on the endocrine system and the maladies of metabolic syndrome, obesity, prediabetes, and type 2 diabetes, I was temporarily flummoxed by the confusing, disjointed, convoluted presentations of these disease states. As I said earlier, it's no wonder that doctors, nurses, and allied health professionals dread working with the endocrine system. I've heard endocrinologists lament, "I don't like to work with patients with type 2 diabetes; they are always overweight and lazy, have no self-control, and never do what I ask of them." (I wonder if they knew I was one of those "darn type 2s"?) Before we knew that type 2 diabetes had genetic and environmental causes, it seemed as if we either got diabetes or we didn't. We now understand the choices we can make to prevent or control it.

But how does one go from making excess insulin and getting fatter to having prediabetes or type 2 diabetes, with the hallmark of high blood sugar? Unlike a body that always responds correctly in regard to the fat-gain hormone insulin, those with Met B are prone to overreact with insulin. As they get fatter, their fat cells literally grow, and their receptors change shape. As time passes, the insulin that is released doesn't fit (a condition known as insulin resistance). The cells continue to scream to be opened and fed, the brain signals the pancreas that it needs more insulin, but insulin keys are not effective. Still more insulin is requested, but this insulin, too, is less effective at opening the cells to remove sugar from the blood. In the meantime, the pancreas is working and working and working—actually overworking—to produce more and more insulin. There comes a time when the pancreas says, "enough," and its insulin-making cells (beta cells) slowly burn out.

At this time, the person has two problems: a fatiguing pancreas and a problem with connecting insulin to the cells (insulin resistance). Blood sugar begins to back up in the bloodstream (causing slightly higher blood sugar readings, or prediabetes), but the cells continue to scream to be fed. If you checked the insulin level for this person, it would most likely be high.

Cravings for carbohydrates worsen, and fatigue, depression, irritability, and malaise sets in as the cells are not being adequately refueled. The liver is continually called upon to release more glycogen stores, the person is craving and consuming more and more carbs, the pancreas is continually in frenzy, and the insulin that is released is not effective.

The state of prediabetes can go on for years—years of feeling awful, getting fatter, and suffering ravenous, insatiable hunger. As time passes, more and more insulin-producing beta cells burn out, and eventually the scales tip: The person moves from having prediabetes to full-blown type 2 diabetes.

If you have type 2 diabetes, your body cannot physiologically produce enough insulin to open an adequate number of cells to fuel the
body. Sugar trapped in the blood rises higher and higher but is literally
stuck in the bloodstream for longer periods of time. Ironically, the person with type 2 diabetes can have high levels of insulin and sugar in
his bloodstream at the same time. Insulin resistance will not allow the
insulin to do its job.

Met B, prediabetes, and type 2 diabetes are all caused by a progressive imbalance of insulin. Uncontrolled Met B causes excess insulin
production, which leads to excess fat storage both on the body and in
the blood. After years of unchecked Met B, prediabetes surfaces when
the pancreas begins to fatigue (producing a little less insulin), and the
insulin becomes less effective (insulin resistance). Over time, uncontrolled prediabetes will ultimately lead to type 2 diabetes, when the
overworked pancreas irreversibly fatigues, producing much less insulin with greater insulin resistance. Type 2 diabetes is not curable,
but it is controllable.

Notice that when I discussed the progression from Met B to prediabetes to type 2 diabetes, that the progression revolves around uncontrolled insulin. If a person was able to control his insulin during the
time he had Met B, could he prevent the onset of prediabetes? The
answer is yes. If a person has already progressed to prediabetes, but he
was able to gain control of his insulin, could he prevent the progression to type 2 diabetes? Again, the answer is yes. If a person progressed
beyond prediabetes to a diagnosis of type 2 diabetes, and he got his
blood sugar under control, is his diabetes gone or reversed? Unfortunately, the answer in this case is no. Diabetes is not reversed or cured,
but his diabetes is under control.

It is possible to control Met B, prediabetes, and diabetes. In each
case, you can be very healthy and avoid complications. Having your
insulin controlled is very good news. You can stop Met B from progressing to prediabetes. You can stop prediabetes from progressing to

type 2 diabetes, but you can't reverse type 2 diabetes, no matter what you might hear or read. Those with type 2 diabetes can, however, keep their blood sugar and weight under control and require the least amount of medication to lead a lean, healthy, happy life.

MEDICATION IS NOT THE ONLY ANSWER

Let's start by telling the facts. Most oral medications that lower blood sugar do so by forcing the pancreas to work even harder and make more and more insulin. (See medications on page 302.) You read that right. Many diabetes medications work by forcing the tired and fatiguing pancreas to work harder to produce enough insulin to drop the blood sugar into the normal range. Over time, this is a damaging scenario because these medications will speed the burn out of the beta cells. This is why people with diabetes who are on oral medications start with one medication, then require two or three, then the doses increase, then they end up injecting insulin.

If it were possible to take some of the stress off the pancreas, you might actually stop this progression. For a moment, let's talk about the other end of the problem, the misshapen insulin receptors that lead to insulin resistance. If we could improve the connection of our own insulin keys to our cells, wouldn't that take some of the pressure off the tired pancreas to produce more and more insulin? The answer is an emphatic yes. (There are some diabetes medications that work to help the connection of insulin keys to cells; metformin is one of them.)

DECREASE INSULIN RESISTANCE WITHOUT MEDICATION

There is a nonmedicinal way to decrease insulin resistance. The name of this method is the Diabetes Miracle (lifestyle program begins on page 113). If fat cells could revert back to their normal size, the connection of insulin to the keyholes (receptors) would improve.

If you were able to promote shrinkage of your overstretched fat cells, the receptors might be able revert to their ideal shape. Terrific — but those of us with Met B, prediabetes, and diabetes can't seem to lose the fat permanently, and the medications we are often prescribed actually force our pancreas to make more insulin, making us even fatter. So, how can a person affect the connection of insulin to the cell without taking a medication?

The answer lies in making dietary and lifestyle changes that work with Met B, rather than against it. The first step is awareness. Jane and Jean are of similar age, weight, and height and have the same fasting lab work. The difference in how they respond to their condition lies in Jean's being made aware of having Met B and Jane's having no idea that her metabolism is working against her.

PATIENT NAME: JANE S.

Year One

Age: 54
Height/Weight: 5 feet, 4 inches, 182 pounds
Gender: Female

Lab Results:
- Glucose: 91 mg/dL (lab reference range: 65–99 mg/dL)
- Triglycerides: 109 mg/dL (lab reference range: under 150 mg/dL)
- LDL cholesterol: 110 mg/dL (lab reference range: under 130 mg/dL)
- A1C: 5.1% (lab reference range: 5.0–5.6 mg/dL)
- Vitamin D: 38 mg/dL (lab reference range: more than 32 mg/dL)

Jane's physician tells her that all her labs are in the normal range, shakes her hand, and schedules her for a physical next year, reminding her to lose weight. Jane spends the year on and off a calorie-based diet and begins to exercise, hoping to look and feel better.

Year Two

Age: 55

Height/Weight: 5 feet, 4 inches, 191 pounds (weight gain of 9 pounds)

Lab Results:

- Glucose: 96 mg/dL (increase)
- Triglycerides: 114 mg/dL (increase)
- LDL cholesterol: 117 mg/dL (increase)
- A1C: 5.3% (increase)
- Vitamin D: 33 mg/dL (decrease)

"Labs still normal, Jane! See you next year . . . remember to work on that weight." Jane is amazed she had actually gained weight even as she'd been much better about dieting and exercising. She decides to try harder and crank up the activity. She could fix this problem. She's grateful to be healthy.

Year Three

Age: 56

Height/Weight: 5 feet, 3 ¾ inches, 193 pounds (height loss of ¼ inch; weight gain of 2 pounds)

Lab Results:

- Glucose: 101 mg/dL (increase)
- Triglycerides: 136 mg/dL (increase)
- LDL cholesterol: 139 mg/dL (increase)
- A1C: 5.7% (increase)
- Vitamin D: 27 mg/dL (decrease)

Jane cringes as she hears, "You gained weight, and now you have prediabetes. Your triglycerides have risen significantly, you have lost one-quarter of an inch in height, and your weight is up 11 pounds in the last two years. Your low vitamin D needs treatment. What happened to you, Jane? Here's a prescription for metformin (to control the amount of glucose in the blood), a statin (to lower cholesterol), and prescription Vitamin D. Consider having a bone density scan and make an appointment with a nutritionist, a cardiologist and an endocrinologist. Let's repeat your labs in three months and hope for the best."

Jane leaves the office in tears. If only she had worked harder, eaten better, and exercised more. Everything was "fine" a year ago.

Patient Name: Jean S.

Year One

Age: 54
Height/Weight: 5 feet, 4 inches, 182 pounds
Gender: Female

Lab Results:
- Glucose: 91 mg/dL (lab reference range: 65–99 mg/dL)
- Triglycerides: 109 mg/dL (lab reference range: under 150 mg/dL)
- LDL cholesterol: 110 mg/dL (lab reference range: under 130 mg/dL)
- A1C: 5.1% (lab reference range: 5.0–5.6%)
- Vitamin D: 38 mg/dL (lab reference range: more than 32 mg/dL)

Jean had been told that although all her lab work was in the medically normal range, her labs indicated that she had Metabolism B. Her physician described the genetic predisposition to insulin imbalance and resistance and suggested she follow the Diabetes Miracle lifestyle. She began the Diabetes Miracle program and returned for her annual physical. At the same time that Jane was told her health and weight required an overhaul and multiple medications, Jean had already lost weight and was maintaining her desired weight of 151 pounds, her lab work remained medically normal, and she needed no medication or specialist consults. She looked great, felt great, and prevented a future of medical woes.

The tale of Jane and Jean plays out every day in physician's offices around the world. Patients who get a heads-up from their health care team can make lifestyle changes that will prevent progressive weight and health woes, help them look and feel great, and potentially change the outcome of their life.

In the next two chapters, you will gain an intimate understanding of prediabetes and type 2 diabetes. Empowered with solid knowledge of these conditions, Chapter 9 then will begin to present the lifestyle program that can control these conditions and help you regain and maintain great health and well-being.

PREDIABETES: YOU CAN REVERSE IT

Larry had to admit that he just didn't feel like himself. He sat in his office with the door uncharacteristically closed. He found himself battling fatigue. One day at 2:00 PM, in the middle of a workday and during the busiest time of the year at the accounting firm, Larry shut his eyes.

He was awakened by the voice of his supervisor: "Larry . . . come on, man, this is the second time this week I've walked in to find you nodding off on the job."

Larry abruptly sat up and realized he had a dull headache that throbbed with his surge in adrenaline. "Sorry, Jim, I didn't sleep well last night. I could not turn my brain off, and before I knew it the alarm was ringing. It won't happen again."

After Jim left, Larry sat quietly. "I have been having difficulty falling asleep lately and I am so tired when it's time to get up. I am sluggish after lunch, and I doze off on the sofa right after dinner. I'm starting to feel a whole lot older than 52. And, honestly, I am starting to look older too. My face is a bit bloated, I have a new double chin, and my belly—how can I have gone from a 36 waist to a 40 (and face it, the 40 is getting tight) in two years?

"Well, it may be because I don't exercise anymore. Work is very stressful, the kids are all involved in sports, and I like to watch them play. I have no time for myself, and when I do, all I want to do is sleep. How did that happen? I used to love to work out.

"In fact, Dr. Lee told me to exercise more, not less! He said I had gained ten pounds in one year, and my blood pressure and cholesterol were on the rise too. He increased my blood pressure medication and started me on a statin to lower cholesterol but reminded me that if I lost some weight, I probably wouldn't need these medications. He also mentioned he's 'watching my sugar,' whatever that meant. Somehow all I managed to do is gain more weight. I'm up four more pounds since I saw Dr. Lee.

"But I am always hungry. If I open a box of crackers, I go back time and again for more. If I start with handful of grapes, I end up finishing the bunch. And forget about ice cream. When I open a container, I feel like it calls my name . . . one scoop, two scoops, three scoops, four. When did I lose my willpower?

"My mom was a lot like I am now. She had type 2 diabetes, though. I hope I do not have diabetes like her. Could I?

"My wife is getting annoyed with me. She says I am irritable and have a very short fuse. I tell her it's because she is always adding to my honey-do list. She's always telling me: 'Larry, you never finish what you start these days. You have started ten projects, but none is finished. You can't seem to focus.'

"Speaking of Joann, I love the woman and really find her attractive, but I have very little interest in sex; the last time we were intimate, I couldn't perform. Maybe that's part of the reason I've been feeling depressed lately."

Larry decided to call Dr. Lee. It was almost time for his annual physical, and he really was feeling like a mess. As he filled out the intake form in the waiting room, he left the section on "what is your chief complaint?" blank. He shook his head as he thought, there are too many to list.

Larry's Symptoms

- Fatigue—especially first thing in the morning and after meals
- Inability to get a good night's sleep or to stay asleep (restless sleep)
- Dull headache around the eyes/sinus area
- Feeling older
- Bloated face, chin
- Weight gain around the middle
- Feeling stressed and anxious at times
- No energy to exercise
- Increased blood pressure
- Elevated cholesterol
- Rising blood sugar
- Constant hunger
- Difficulty in stopping eating carbohydrates
- Family history of type 2 diabetes
- Irritability, a short fuse
- Mild depression
- Low libido and erectile dysfunction

Fortunately, Dr. Lee recognized Larry's multitude of symptoms as those of uncontrolled Met B. He ordered several blood tests and confirmed that Larry did, indeed, have prediabetes. This was lucky for Larry. Another physician might assume Larry was getting older, had young children that wore him out, and was working hard to make ends meet. Larry could follow the Diabetes Miracle and correct the metabolic mayhem while improving his health and quality of life.

THE GIFT OF A PREDIABETES DIAGNOSIS

If I told you that the diagnosis of prediabetes was a gift, you'd probably think I was crazy. Anything involving diabetes has to be bad, right? Prediabetes can be considered the gray zone between normal blood sugar and type 2 diabetes. The actual diagnosis of prediabetes is based on the results of a fasting glucose test, oral glucose tolerance test, or hemoglobin A1C level. The diagnosis is made when you have a fasting blood sugar of 100–125 mg/dL or HbA1C of 5.7–6.4 percent. Most people diagnosed with prediabetes progress to type 2 diabetes in less than ten years. Prediabetes has also been called borderline diabetes, impaired fasting blood glucose, impaired glucose tolerance, or a "touch" of diabetes. The term prediabetes appears to be the best term for the condition, as it gives a clear picture of what is transpiring in the body—the calm before the potential storm of type 2 diabetes. If a person with prediabetes makes the proper lifestyle changes, he can prevent or greatly delay the onset of irreversible type 2 diabetes and can be healthier and happier than he ever imagined possible.

Not so many years ago, there was no definitive diagnosis of prediabetes. The diagnosis of diabetes was made at a much higher benchmark. In many cases, type 2 diabetes wasn't diagnosed until blood sugar exceeded 200 mg/dL and showed up in the urine. Back in the day, if blood sugar was elevated, patients were informed that their blood sugar was "creeping up" or that they had a "touch of sugar." We now know that based on a fasting blood glucose reading of more than 200 mg/dL, the patients with a "touch of sugar" already had diabetes.

TOO SWEET FOR YOUR OWN GOOD

Prediabetes usually arrives with a posse of companions, including weight around the middle, rising blood pressure, and elevated LDL cholesterol, triglycerides, and blood sugar. When your fasting blood sugar exceeds 99 mg/dL, your health care provider should pay close attention to these other health markers because your risk for heart attack and stroke is higher than normal when your blood sugar is elevated.

ADDITIONAL RISKS

A person with prediabetes has a one and a half times higher risk for cardiovascular disease than those without prediabetes.

A person with type 2 diabetes has a two times higher risk of heart attack or stroke than she would have if she did not have diabetes.

Why would a slight increase in blood sugar make such a dire difference in cardiovascular risk? When you metabolically arrive at prediabetes, your blood is averaging higher than the normal, but not as high as in the diagnosis of diabetes.

A higher concentration of sugar in the blood makes the blood "stickier" than normal. The sticky consistency of this blood makes it the perfect medium for enabling excess fatty components, such as LDL cholesterol and triglycerides, to adhere to the blood vessel's wall and become "glued" to the inner walls of the vessel. Hence, a person with prediabetes has a built-in medium for building plaque deposits at a faster rate because the sticky walls automatically latch onto passing minerals, cholesterol, and triglycerides. The old image of hardening of the arteries is a picturesque way to describe the stiff artery walls that are the result of years of hardened high sugar and lipids within the arteries. The vessel's pliability diminishes, and the vessels become less flexible.

Over time, the interior diameter of the blood vessel narrows from the excessive fat deposits. The pressure of blood pumped through narrowed vessel walls increases. This high pressure within the blood vessels is hypertension (high blood pressure). Narrower blood vessels leave less room for passage, and a person with a history of high blood sugar runs the risk of a heart attack or stroke from a clot that lodges in the narrowed or blocked vessel.

INFLAMMATION

Some physicians have begun routinely to order a lab test called C-reactive protein (CRP), which measures inflammation. CRP is a reactant released by the body in response to acute injury, infection, and fever and indicates a heightened state of inflammation in the body. Inflammation can damage the inner lining of arteries, causing cracks and crevices that can snag clots and potentially block the flow of blood, triggering strokes and heart attacks.

CRP levels increase with aging, high blood pressure, low levels of physical activity, chronic fatigue, elevated triglycerides, insulin resistance, diabetes, sleep disturbances, and depression. These are all also the subclinical symptoms of Met B. Alcohol and caffeine can also elevate CRP. You may consider requesting a routine CRP to be added to routine lab work as another indicator of possible Met B.

INFLAMMATION AND DIABETES

Inflammation is the body's response to injury. When inflammation occurs, the body sends cells to destroy or remove damaged tissue. There is a link between inflammation and diabetes. For years, inflammation was linked to heart disease, but now it appears to play a role in the development of diabetes also.

There are blood tests to show markers for inflammation in the bloodstream (inflammatory activity). One of these markers, C-reactive protein (CRP), is best known as an indicator of heart disease or heart attack. Now, elevated CRP has been linked to obesity, type 2 diabetes, and heart disease. *

---

*American Diabetes Association, "Inflammation and Type 2 Diabetes," *ADA Meeting Report*, June 16, 2002.

LOSING (SOME) WEIGHT

Although there is no magic pill for treating prediabetes, there are definitely things you can do. Fortunately, the treatment consists of lifestyle changes: specifically losing weight and engaging in more physical activity. Even a modest weight loss of ten to fifteen pounds can make a big difference in fighting diabetes. Moderate exercise, such as walking thirty minutes a day five days a week, can help regulate blood sugar.

Unfortunately, many people step on a scale, see that they are seventy-five pounds above what their weight should be as shown on the "ideal body weight chart," and throw in the towel. Granted, losing seventy-five pounds can seem like a daunting challenge, especially for someone who has always had difficulty losing weight because of the insulin issues that accompany uncontrolled Met B.

We now know that you needn't reach your ideal body weight to see great results in blood sugar, and a ten- to fifteen-pound loss of fat will make a tremendous difference in how your body handles blood sugar. Think of weight loss as a long-term project. It didn't take eight weeks to gain that weight, so it will not take eight weeks to lose it.

DON'T BELIEVE WEIGHT CHARTS

I have a private practice in medical nutrition therapy and have been a registered dietitian and diabetes specialist for many years. I do not use height/weight charts or figure body mass index (BMI) in my practice. I choose not to use them because I have seen time and time again that the number on a scale reveals very little about the health status of the individual.

I have two female patients, Sharon and Caroline. Sharon is 55 years of age; Caroline is 25. Both are 5 feet 5 inches and weigh 150 pounds. If I were using height/weight charts, I would use their gender, height, and present weight to determine if they are underweight, normal weight, or overweight. Both Caroline and Sharon would be told they are overweight because the chart lists their normal body weight as 113–138 pounds. I should mention that Sharon has prediabetes, hypertension, low HDL cholesterol, high LDL cholesterol, and a roll of fat around her tummy. She does not regularly exercise, takes medication for blood pressure and cholesterol, and wears a clothing size that she dislikes. It is no surprise that she is at an unhealthy weight.

But what about Caroline? If I were using height/weight charts, I would have to tell the 25-year-old that she is overweight. But at the same height and weight as Sharon, Caroline looks much different. Did I mention that Caroline is a marathon runner? She fits into a much smaller clothing size; runs daily; feels great; and has normal blood sugar, blood pressure, and cholesterol. She takes no medication and is the picture of health. But according to those charts, she's overweight.

Because of weight charts, both women are concerned about their weight. Caroline feels that she looks great, feels great, and has great lab work and blood pressure, but her primary doctor keeps telling her she needs to lose weight. Sharon has medical conditions that already require medication, is larger than she wants to be, dislikes how she looks, and is often fatigued and unhappy.

Remember that these charts only factor in gender, height, and weight. They do not take into account body frame, bone density, muscle mass, age, or activity level. Caroline was thrilled to hear this explanation, and Sharon realized it wasn't the number on the scale that was the issue; it was her health and body image at her present weight.

DO NOT BELIEVE IN BMI

Maybe because height/weight charts aren't so helpful, the buzz word in dieting has become "BMI." Many magazines and weight-loss programs, and even your physician, may assume BMI is a more accurate way to determine healthy weight than weight-loss charts. Unfortunately, BMI is no better measure of ideal weight than the old height/weight charts. BMI is determined by multiplying your weight by your height, squared. Not to worry—there are tables everywhere that do the math for you. The normal range of BMI is within 18.5 and 24.9. Anything under 18.5 is labeled underweight on the body mass index. The overweight BMI range is between 25 and 29.9. You are considered obese if your BMI is more than 30. You are morbidly obese if your BMI is more than 40. BMI takes into account two things only: height and weight. There is not even a different BMI for gender, so men and women use the same BMI formula. BMI, like the height and weight charts, does not factor in gender, body frame, bone density, muscle mass, age, or physical activity.

Phil is a 25-year-old male athlete who is 5 feet 6 inches and weighs 170 pounds. He has a large frame, perfect bone density, and a lot of muscle. His BMI is 27.4. His physician classified him as overweight, according to BMI measures.

Jillian is a 70-year-old retired librarian and is now sedentary. She is 5 feet 6 inches and weighs 170 pounds. She is small-boned, has been told she has declining bone density, and has much more fat than muscle mass. Her BMI is 27.4. She is also overweight per her BMI.

Phil is lean, healthy, looks great, and is in top physical condition. He is happy with how he looks and feels, all his health parameters are normal, and he takes no medication.

Jillian has high body fat (especially around the middle); is in extra-large clothing; and has prediabetes, hypertension, and high cholesterol. She keeps track of multiple medications by using a daily pill box. She feels too fatigued to exercise. She is very unhappy with the way she looks.

When you really understand what height/weight charts and BMI don't measure, you can see that using them to determine a healthy weight or whether or not you are overweight is pointless: They tell us nothing valuable.

KEEPING TRACK OF IDEAL BODY WEIGHT—WITHOUT A SCALE

1. Keep a running log of your Met B–related fasting lab work (see page 340 for a sample form). Keep track of your labs and look for trends. You always want to see labs as near to normal as possible on as little medication as possible.
2. Keep an updated list of medications and doses. Make a notation if dosages increase or decrease. It's best to use medications at the smallest possible doses to keep your body functioning in a healthy way. Don't let "normal labs" fool you if they are brought about by overmedication.
3. Pay attention to your clothing size. Next to your labs, make note of the size of your shirts and slacks. Keep a running track: neck measurement, shirts, jeans, slacks, and dresses.
4. Consider keeping and rechecking body measurements every eight weeks (see page 335 for body measurement sheet). Keep a running track of them.
5. Take a picture. I often recommend that my patients take a picture of themselves in a particular form-fitting outfit at the start of every eight-week period. Sometimes the mind's eye does not let you appreciate the tremendous progress you are making in reshaping and taking control of your weight and health. When you objectively look at pictures of yourself in the same outfit side by side every eight weeks, there is no mistaking it. The picture will show you what your mind may not allow you to see.

DETERMINING A HEALTHY WEIGHT

Determining what is healthiest for your body is not as simple as using the number on a scale and comparing it to ranges on a chart. As a medical nutrition specialist, I consider ideal body weight to be the scale weight at which the individual requires as little medication as possible, has normal nutritionally related lab values and blood pressure, is satisfied with the way her body looks and feels, and is wearing the size clothes she desires. She should feel great too. To me, this is a person's ideal body weight.

Gradually, you will reach the weight at which you need little or no medication, your labs are normal, you look great, and you feel great. Voilà . . . the number on the scale that matches your healthy body is your ideal body weight.

EXERCISE

Aside from losing some weight (remember, as little as ten pounds can make a big difference), another way to help stop the progression of prediabetes to type 2 diabetes is to become physically active. Thankfully, you needn't become a marathon runner, gym rat, or fitness guru.

Assess what your level of normal physical activity is right now, and move your body an additional thirty minutes a day. If you are not exercising at all, you can consider adding thirty minutes of walking into your day: ten minutes in the morning, ten in the afternoon, and ten in the evening. If you are already walking thirty minutes a day three days per week, consider increasing to five days a week. If you have a physical job, such as shelf stocking, hands-on nursing, or construction, you can consider adding something fun—shooting hoops, riding a bicycle, or even engaging in daily yoga to change it up and move different muscles. The good news is that you do not need to do thirty minutes of increased activity all in one shot. You can spread it out throughout the day. It all counts.

WHEN SHOULD I EXERCISE?

The best time to exercise for someone with Met B is within one to two hours after the start of a meal, when blood sugar is most likely at its highest. Exercised muscles will uptake blood sugar from the meal for energy. Even after exercise, sensitized muscles will attract insulin, diverting these keys from opening fat cells. Exercising after eating also helps decrease the chance for low blood sugar.

If you prefer to exercise before breakfast, make sure to eat an appropriate snack prior to working out. This snack will suppress the liver's self-feeding mechanism that engaged while you were sleeping. If you exercise in the morning without shutting down the liver glycogen release, your insulin will overrelease during exercise. Then you can actually gain fat and may see a rise in blood sugar from exercise. Ironically, if you exercise in the morning without a pre-exercise snack, it can slow weight loss and increase blood sugar.

FREQUENCY OF EXERCISE TRUMPS DURATION OF EXERCISE

It is much more beneficial to exercise five days of the week for thirty minutes than two days of the week for ninety minutes each day. Exercise that burns blood sugar on a daily basis will decrease your blood sugar and the need for sugar-lowering medication. Muscle movement will increase blood sugar uptake (by the energized muscle tissue) for hours afterward.

You can divide your exercise to keep sugar uptake high throughout the day. Fifteen minutes in the morning briskly walking the dog and fifteen minutes in the evening walking around the neighborhood, or ten minutes at three different times during the day, will all be effective. You can also exercise for more than thirty minutes on any given day. (See the Fueling It Forward Exercise on page 176.) The idea is to move your muscles a minimum of thirty minutes a day, five times per week, over and above their normal activity.

For much more on exercise, see Chapter 12 (page 245).

LARRY GOES TO THE DOCTOR AND MAKES SOME CHANGES

Larry's visit to his doctor was a life-changer. Dr. Lee recommended the lifestyle program that is in *The Diabetes Miracle* and suggested Larry return in eight weeks for follow-up lab work. Larry was surprised that he did not add or increase any medications, but Dr. Lee told him that he wanted to revisit his weight and labs after he "detoxed." Unsure of what he meant, Larry began the program.

The lab work Dr. Lee ordered for Larry (height 5 feet 9 inches, weight 210 pounds) based on his plethora of symptoms is as follows:

- Metabolic panel
- Lipid Profile
- Hemoglobin A1C
- Vitamin D.

Larry was instructed to take body measurements at home and repeat after eight weeks. Larry used the format in *The Diabetes Miracle* to keep track of his weight and measurements.

Larry read the Diabetes Miracle lifestyle program (included here) twice and went to work on changing his lifestyle as described. Eight weeks later, he returned to Dr. Lee's office, looking and feeling like a new man.

Below are a before and after look at Larry's lab work as it pertains to Met B:

Test (normal range)	Start value	After 8 weeks
Glucose: (65–89 mg/dL)	117mg/dL	102 mg/dL
Total chol: (under 200 mg/dL)	217 mg/dL	193 mg/dL
LDL chol: (under 130 mg/dL)	137 mg/dL	95 mg/dL
HDL chol: (greater than 45 mg/dL)	36 mg/dL	42 mg/dL
Triglycerides (under 150 mg/dL)	145 mg/dL	110 mg/dL
A1C (5.3–5.6%)	5.9 mg/dL	5.6 mg/dL
Vitamin D (greater than 32 mg/dL)	26 mg/dL	36 mg/dL

Weight: lost 10 pounds (within expected loss of 6–13 pounds)
Total inches lost: 12 (within expected inch loss of 11–13 inches)

Dr. Lee was thrilled with the improvement in Larry's weight, inches lost, and all his Met B–related labs. He advised him to move on to Step 2 and return in three months for a follow-up, at which time he would revisit his weight loss, inches lost, and labs. Larry got the feeling that if things continued to improve, he wouldn't be adding medication; he'd be decreasing it.

Larry also told Dr. Lee about the tremendous change in his quality of life. He had energy to spare, was starting and finishing jobs, excelled at work, was not short-tempered, and felt that his depression had abated. Life was good, and Larry felt reborn.

Larry was able, through diet and exercise, to stop the progression from prediabetes to type 2 diabetes. If you already have been diagnosed with type 2 diabetes, don't despair—understanding your disease and its health risks can help you to effectively make changes to improve your health outcomes.

TYPE 2 DIABETES:
YOU CAN CONTROL IT

If nothing is done to moderate blood sugar and resultant insulin release, the pancreas's insulin-producing beta cells fatigue, and the insulin produced is not sufficient to moderate blood sugar peaks. As a result, fasting blood sugar levels will exceed 125 mg/dL and hemoglobin A1C will exceed 6.4. The person with prediabetes now has been diagnosed with type 2 diabetes.

Once you cross the line to type 2 diabetes, you will always have type 2 diabetes. Your aim should be to keep type 2 diabetes under excellent control on as little medication as possible so you can lead a long, healthy, happy life. Through diet and exercise, a person with type 2 diabetes can live a lifestyle to produce a normal amount of blood sugar that the pancreas can reasonably handle. Some people can attain blood glucose control with a combination of diet and exercise whereas others require diet, exercise, and medication.

Although you initially may be prescribed medication to control blood sugar, by making and maintaining necessary lifestyle changes, it is possible that you will no longer require diabetes medication. It is not true that once you begin medication for type 2 diabetes, you can never get off of it. It is not true that once you start insulin therapy for type 2 diabetes, you will always require it. It is not true that if you live long enough with diabetes, you will require insulin. No matter what medication you are taking or how much, you can help your cause along by living a life that matches your present metabolic state.

THE ROOT OF THE PROBLEM

Diabetes is a disease with genetic roots. A person is born with the genetic propensity to develop type 2 diabetes. If a person does not have the genes for type 2 diabetes, he has little chance of developing type 2 diabetes. If a person with textbook metabolism (no insulin imbalance) gains weight, doesn't exercise, and doesn't eat appropriately, he won't necessarily develop diabetes because he doesn't have the genes to support diabetes. This is why you will find that some people are heavier, less active, and less food-conscious than you but do not have diabetes. The truth of the matter is that your genetic blueprint set you up with the potential to develop diabetes, and a progressive hormonal imbalance pushed along by environmental triggers silently battered at your metabolism for years before your blood sugar rose to the level that brought on the diagnosis.

Many people diagnosed with diabetes are in denial, thinking, "No one in my family has or has had diabetes." Even though you may not be aware of it, yes, they did or do have it or will develop it. Because of the way diabetes was diagnosed in the past, it is possible that you didn't know that your parents, grandparents, or great grandparents really did have undiagnosed diabetes because they themselves did not know.

Currently, diabetes is diagnosed when fasting blood sugar exceeds 125 mg/dL. Not so long ago, the diagnosis of diabetes was not made until blood sugar was measured at closer to 200 mg/dL. As a result, many people who really had diabetes were never diagnosed. They had the subclinical symptoms of fatigue, irritability, carbohydrate cravings, blurry vision, and inability to focus or concentrate. They also most likely had the accompanying medical conditions of hypertension, high cholesterol, and midline fat. Their family had a medical history of heart attacks or strokes. But because their blood sugar was not high enough to qualify as diabetes, they were never diagnosed.

Also, there may be members of your family tree who have type 2 diabetes right now and are simply unaware. The common, publicized symptoms of diabetes—excessive thirst, urination, hunger, and blurry vision—usually don't occur until blood sugar regularly exceeds 200 mg/dL. It can take years of disease progression for diabetes to cause blood sugars that regularly exceed 200 mg/dL and cause these well-known symptoms. Because some people don't get annual physical exams and only visit their physician if they have a medical problem, they can live with undiagnosed and untreated diabetes for years. Your parents, grandparents, aunts, uncles, cousins, and even your children may have undiagnosed diabetes.

Now that you know that you have prediabetes or type 2 diabetes, and you are aware that it is genetically passed, it's important to be aware that members of your family might be in line to develop type 2 diabetes. The good news is that you can inform your family of your diagnosis so they can have an opportunity to determine if they, too, have Metabolism B, prediabetes, or type 2 diabetes as well as the opportunity to prevent the progression to diabetes by getting the condition under control as soon as possible.

BOARDING THE DIABETES TRAIN

Type 2 diabetes does not normally happen overnight; it is a progressive disease. The potential for developing type 2 actually begins at the time of a person's birth. At that time, the newborn already has the genetic makeup to make the disease possible. Think of it like boarding a train. Because of genetic inheritance (the ticket), some people get on the A train and will always have normal regulation of blood sugar, and some people will get on the B train (Met B) and will always be at risk for developing abnormal blood sugar. The B train moves along the tracks toward type 2 diabetes, picking up speed to full-blown diabetes because of life's stressors.

LIFE'S STRESSORS PROVIDE MORE FUEL FOR THE DIABETES TRAIN

It appears that life's stressors contribute to the speed at which the diabetes train runs. The more stressors a person with Met B experiences, the faster type 2 diabetes develops.

Weight gain. When a person gains weight, it's easy to see the increased size of fat deposits on her body: a fatter belly, love handles, muffin top, and back fat are all descriptions of getting fatter. As a person gets fatter, she is not producing additional fat cells; rather, the fat cells she already has are increasing in size. The larger fat cells become, the less effective insulin becomes. Insulin resistance means there is plenty, probably excess, insulin in the blood, but it is not working effectively. As a result, the overworking pancreas is asked to make more and more insulin in an attempt to regulate blood sugar. The fatter a person with uncontrolled Met B becomes, the greater the insulin resistance, and the faster her progression to diabetes.

Normal hormonal changes. A person's body undergoes normal hormonal changes throughout his lifetime. At puberty, there is an increase in sex or reproductive hormones. Often right around the time of puberty, there is a growth spurt that requires a surge in growth hormone. A common time for symptoms of Met B to emerge (for both sexes) is between the ages of 18 to 23. Another normal hormonal change occurs during pregnancy and lactation, when hormonal levels undergo tremendous swings. It's not a coincidence that many women first notice symptoms of uncontrolled Met B after the birth of a child.

There is also great hormonal flux in the years before, during, or after menopause. The aging process itself causes hormonal change. Whenever hormonal levels make a significant rise or fall, the Met B train gets extra fuel as it lumbers down the tracks toward type 2 diabetes.

Smoking. If you smoke, you need to quit. Smoking increases your risk of diabetes complications, including heart attack, stroke, nerve damage, and kidney disease. Smokers with diabetes are three times more likely to die of a heart attack or stroke than diabetics who don't smoke, according to the ADA.* The chances of suffering a cardiovascular death are much too high when you have diabetes and smoke.

Stress. When a person experiences stress, a small region at the base of the brain called the hypothalamus sets off an alarm throughout the body. The alarm prompts the adrenal glands (located at the top of the kidneys) to release stress hormones, such as cortisol, adrenaline, and epinephrine. One of the main functions of stress hormones is to prompt a quick rise in blood sugar to fuel the fight-or-flight response. This response is built into human physiology to deliver a surge of energy when a person needs to run from danger or physically defend himself. This surge was especially necessary and beneficial in the past when people had to physically fight to survive or had to run from invaders for safety. As blood sugar spiked, the person had instantaneous fuel to run or fight. The act of running or fighting burned off the excess blood sugar, and in the end, there was blood sugar equilibrium.

Today's stress is much different than fighting a pack of invaders or running from a wild animal. In many people's everyday life, a combination of stressors leaves them feeling anxious, tense, on edge, and irritable. Today's stressors may include the economic picture, a demanding

---

*www.vahealth.org/cdpc/TUCP/documents/2011/pdf/StateFact_Sheets/Smoking%20and%20Diabetes.pdf.

Dealing with Stress
in the Modern World

Because we don't typically respond to stress with the physical activity of fight or flight, regular physical activity is important to burn excess blood sugar produced by daily stressors.

boss, difficulty paying the mortgage or day-to-day bills, marriages and children, elder care, commuting, and on and on. Unfortunately, we can't always physically fight our way out of or actually run away from daily chronic stress, and our blood sugar and insulin release remain in high gear.

The blood sugar spikes and insulin release caused by chronic stress in the twenty-first century are ever present. The longer or more intense the stress, the higher the blood sugar spikes, the more insulin releases, the fatter a person becomes, the more the insulin receptors change shape, the faster the pancreas tires, and the faster the train speeds toward type 2 diabetes.

Illness and healing. When a person is ill, her body works to heal itself. Hormones such as cortisol, DHEA, human growth hormone, melatonin, and serotonin are all involved in healing and wellness. These healing and wellness hormones raise blood sugar to provide energy for the healing process. The longer or more ill a person is, the longer and higher the blood sugar will elevate. The pancreas must respond with more insulin. Prolonged or chronic illness speeds up the fatigue of the pancreas and hastens the progression of Met B to type 2 diabetes. It is often following an illness that a person is diagnosed with type 2 diabetes.

A Personal Story

Last year, when I went for my routine lab work, I was surprised to get a call from my internist telling me that two of my lab results were out of the normal range. My fasting glucose was 128 mg/dL, and my hemoglobin A1C was 6.6.

He was not calling to diagnose diabetes (I've had diabetes for fifteen years); he was calling to tell me that my labs, which I typically maintain in the normal range through lifestyle (diet and exercise), had increased. Before he hung up, he told me he was pleased with all the other results because they were considered "very good" for someone with diabetes. The glucose and HbA1c results were quite unusual for me, and I got off the phone thinking, "What could be going on?"

I hung up with the doctor and went to the mailbox to find the copy of my lab work waiting for me. Although my doctor had reported the increase in glucose and hemoglobin A1C, he had failed to mention that my triglycerides were 134 (for years they had been under 100), my LDL cholesterol was 102 (it has been significantly under 100 for years), and my vitamin D was now deficient (it had been a respectable 48–55 for years).

If I hadn't seen a copy of my labs, I would not have known that my triglycerides, LDL cholesterol, and vitamin D were off base and needed attention.

How did this happen? As I gave the situation some thought, I realized I had been sick (stomach virus followed by a urinary tract infection) and had been under a great deal of stress during the months preceding my lab work. I am fairly certain that the back-to-back illnesses, requiring a course of antibiotics, and the stress in my life caused my lab work to backslide.

Because I check my blood sugar at least twice a day, I knew that my home readings were normal the past few months, albeit a bit higher than usual for me. I attributed their slight increase to illness and stress. The rise in A1C meant that my blood sugar had to be spiking at times other than fasting and two hours post-meals. This is common in illness and during stressful situations. What surprised me was the extent of backsliding that occurred in my overall health picture from stressors that were out of my control.

I immediately began Step 1 of the Diabetes Miracle lifestyle to reset my metabolism and continued my exercise regimen. I had the labs repeated in three months instead of six, and they were back to normal. Although it is important to realize how illness can affect your lab work, this story is also an example of how important it is to ask for a copy of your own blood work and to question changes in your Met B–related labs if they are not mentioned. Both you and your doctor need to be aware of the big picture as it relates to diabetes. Diabetes affects so many aspects of health and well-being, and if you know the whole situation, you are empowered to fix it.

Inactivity. Physical activity and exercise cause muscles to uptake blood sugar for fuel. When muscles consume blood sugar for the purpose of movement and work, blood sugar AND the need for insulin decrease, and the pancreas is less taxed. Also, the act of exercise depletes the muscles' own glycogen stores. With glycogen depleted, the muscles will signal for insulin when it is released after the next meal or snack. Insulin will preferentially help to refill muscles with sugar *before* it moves on to open fat cells.

A sedentary person whose muscles are not activated by movement will maintain higher levels of glucose in the blood, require more insulin production to handle the higher blood sugar, and send the excess insulin keys to open fat cells. Being inactive hastens the progression of uncontrolled Met B to prediabetes to type 2 diabetes.

Pain and inflammation. Pain and inflammation cause the release of stress hormones that cause blood sugar to rise. Many people suffer from chronic pain due to arthritis, recurrent headaches, neuralgia, fibromyalgia, or back problems. Their body's reaction to pain and inflammation causes constant, long-term release of stress hormones, which ultimately hastens pancreas fatigue and the onset of type 2 diabetes. Metabolic syndrome, prediabetes, and type 2 diabetes are now considered to be inflammatory conditions in and of themselves.*

Certain medications. During a person's lifetime, he may be prescribed medications that have adverse effects on blood sugar. A partial list of medications that may cause a rise in blood sugar includes:

- Oral contraceptive agents that contain high levels of estrogen
- Phenytoin or Dilantin (antiepileptics)
- Cortisol or steroids, including cortisone-based skin preparations

---

Nutrition Review 65, no. 2 (December 2007): S152–156.

- Antihypertensives used to lower blood pressure, including: (1) diuretics, such as Diuril, hydrochlorothiazide, Amizide, and Chlotride; (2) beta blockers, such as Inderal, Lopressor, Visken, and Tenormin; and (3) calcium channel blockers, such as Adalat, Cardizem, and Verapamil
- Nicotinic acid, used to lower cholesterol levels
- Estrogen used in hormone replacement therapy during menopause
- Over-the-counter medications, including decongestants containing pseudoephedrine, which alter the level of various hormones responsible for raising blood sugar
- Even caffeine can cause a quick spike in blood sugar within an hour of ingestion. Caffeine is also an added ingredient in some medications.

TAKING MEDICATIONS WITH AWARENESS

When it comes to taking medication, it is often a matter of risk versus benefit. For example, if a person has worsening pneumonia that is not responding to antibiotics, the use of a prednisone-based medication may help get the infection under control. There are times in your life when medication may be needed, although it has a side effect that causes an elevation in blood sugar. During these times, you may *temporarily* require more medication (even insulin) to control blood sugar. Those who take oral medications often require insulin injections during hospitalizations. This is usually temporary, and most of these same people are released home on their oral medication.

Always remind your physician that you have diabetes when she is considering medication choices. It is possible that there may be an alternative medication that won't interfere with blood sugar. In fact, it's a great idea to keep a medication list with dosage in your purse or wallet to show your doctor when new medications are added in case there are potential contraindications or medication interactions.

THE PERFECT STORM:
GENES AND STRESSORS COMBINE

The more life stressors a person with Met B experiences, and the earlier the age of the accumulation of stressors, the younger and faster they can expect to develop type 2 diabetes.

Tom is a 62-year-old overweight man with prediabetes who is currently taking prednisone for pneumonia. When he was in a car accident in which he broke his leg and was unable to exercise at his gym, there would be an excellent chance that he would tremendously speed up his Met B train ride with a final destination of type 2 diabetes.

- Risk factors: age, overweight, and has prediabetes
- Stressors: pneumonia (illness), accident (emotional stress), injury (broken leg), pain and inflammation, decreased mobility (no exercise)
- Medication: steroidal-based prednisone (can elevate blood sugar)

Tom is caught in the perfect storm to develop type 2 diabetes if he has the genetic predisposition.

What can Tom do to avoid progressing from prediabetes to type 2 diabetes during this time of high stress? The best place for Tom to put himself is Step 1 of the Diabetes Miracle. In Step 1, he will control his carbohydrate intake, and his liver will be depleted of glycogen stores. He can also ask his doctor if she can prescribe physical therapy to permit physical activity given his current condition.

COMPLICATIONS FROM
UNCONTROLLED DIABETES

Complications from diabetes come in two varieties: the type that decrease your daily quality of life and those that affect your long-term health. The daily complications are seldom, if ever, mentioned when you read about type 2 diabetes.

DAILY COMPLICATIONS

The daily complications can have a dramatic impact on your quality of life, relationships, self-esteem, safety, how you function in the work-place, and much more.

- Chronic fatigue; waking up tired; and falling asleep or getting woozy driving to work, during meetings, in the late afternoon, or right after dinner
- Craving carbohydrates: the urge, need, or overwhelming desire to eat something you know is not in your best interest, such as chips, pretzels, bread, ice cream, pasta, cookies, or candy
- Poor short-term memory, difficulty focusing, difficulty remembering, racing thoughts, or brain fog
- Short temper, irritability, short fuse, anxiety, panic attacks
- Mild depression, lack of motivation, lack of energy
- Sleep problems, such as sleep apnea or restless sleep; and difficulty falling asleep, staying asleep, or falling back to sleep
- Very easy weight gain, especially around the middle and back (apple shape)
- Increasing generalized aches/pains, joint pain and stiffness, headaches
- Alcohol causes flushing, red cheeks, sweats, light-headedness
- Caffeine has less of an effect
- Decreased libido, erectile dysfunction, yeast infections, lack of energy to initiate sex
- Blurry vision, night driving problems, light sensitivity, teary eyes, dry eyes.

Can you imagine how much more difficult a day is when a person is fatigued; is craving sweets; has no ability to focus and has decreased short-term memory; and is irritable, anxious, and depressed? What if this person hadn't slept well and his joints were stiff and achy? Add to that blurry vision, no energy lift from his daily coffee, and no desire for sex. This is definitely an example of unnecessarily complicated life. Lift these symptoms, and life would be a whole lot easier and much more enjoyable.

These symptoms begin from the time a person's labs indicate Met B, years before the diagnosis of diabetes. The longer a person has *un-controlled* Met B, prediabetes, or type 2 diabetes, the worse the symptoms become.

LONG-TERM COMPLICATIONS

The most notable complications of type 2 diabetes involve high blood sugar that has damaged the body over a period of time. Most people think of the complications of diabetes as blindness, kidney disorders, and poor blood circulation that can lead to amputations, heart attacks, and strokes. After reading this section, my hope is that you will understand how elevated blood sugar can irreversibly damage every blood vessel and nerve in the body and that you will understand that you have the ability and power to take control of your blood sugar TODAY to halt any future damage.

Blood sugar of 65–99 mg/dL is typically the normal range for fasting blood sugar. Blood sugar drawn two hours after the start of a meal doesn't normally exceed 140 mg/dL. Normal hormonal regulation of insulin/glucagon does a wonderful job keeping blood sugar very close to the parameters of this ideal range. Most people with normal blood sugar have readings around 80–125 mg/dL throughout the day. A person with diabetes can have blood sugar that regularly exceeds 140, and can easily exceed 200 mg/dL.

I tell my patients that blood sugar is just what it sounds like: It *is* sugar in the blood. When people prick their finger to test their sugar, they sometimes visualize that their sugar is elevated in that one droplet of blood. I always remind them that when their one droplet of blood shows excess sugar content, every droplet of blood coursing through their veins has elevated sugar content.

Normal blood usually appears fluid-like and bright red in color. Blood with higher sugar appears darker in color and thicker in consistency. When I test my blood sugar and it is elevated, I can see that my reading will be above the normal range by the blood's dark purple color and the relative thickness of the blood sample, though I may not be able to pinpoint the exact reading number. The higher the reading will be, the more syrupy the consistency of the blood droplet. If you place a droplet of highly concentrated blood on a hard surface, you can literally chip it away when it hardens (much the same as you would have to scrape spilled and hardened pancake syrup off of a countertop surface).

It is this sticky, syrupy, sugar-laden blood that causes the long-term damage associated with high blood sugar. Every long-term complication of diabetes can be traced to hardening of vessels, nerves, and tissues from long-term exposure to high concentrations of sugar.

To better understand this concept, try to visualize the making of a candy apple. Dip the apple into melted, liquid sugary syrup. The sticky syrup coats the surface of the apple. Let the apple stand for a bit, and the liquid coating hardens into a crystalline covering that becomes hard to the touch and will actually shatter when you bite into it. If you roll the apple in coconut flakes while the coating is still liquid, the coconut will harden into the syrup and stick as if it were glued to the apple.

Now, visualize the inner lining of your blood vessels as it gets coated with sugary syrup when your blood sugar rises over the normal range. As your heart pumps the sugar-dense blood through every blood vessel, the vessel's lining becomes coated with a syrupy layer. Next, imagine that excesses of cholesterol and triglycerides travel through the very same vessels. These fatty globules will have a perfect sticky medium to adhere to. As time passes, the sticky coating hardens, encasing the cholesterol and triglycerides in its grip. Throughout a day of high blood sugar readings, the process happens over and over again on a microscopic level. Day after day, the layers of syrup harden. Eventually, the blood vessel loses its pliability and becomes hardened and stiff. Blood pressure increases. Over time, the diameter of the inner lining of the vessel is minimized by the thickly coated walls. Not only is there less room for blood to flow, but the hardening and crystallization of the vessels increases the possibility of tiny cracks, rough surfaces, and even built-up blockages that can snag a passing blot clot. Circulation lessens as the vessels become less able to get blood to its destination. The vessels become inflamed.

The same internal sugar coating that occurs inside blood vessels also affects your nerves and nerve endings. The nerves send electrical impulses and messages from the brain to other areas of the body and back. As time passes, this crystallization sugarcoats the nerve endings and impedes the proper flow of nerve conduction. As a result, people with a long-term history of high blood sugar have *hyper*sensitivity or *hypo*sensitivity—either too much or too little sensation.

To give you some idea as to how much actual sugar is contained in elevated blood sugar, I now guesstimate that for every point a person decreases his A1C (lowering the sugar traveling in his blood), he has the potential to gain 5 pounds of weight. If you begin the Diabetes Miracle program with an A1C of 8.5 and make diet, exercise, and medication changes to drop your A1C to a more healthful 6.5, you will have produced a potential 10 pounds fat gain on your body. (Thankfully, the Diabetes Miracle is designed to be a fat-burning diet. As quickly as the fat from excess blood sugar is produced, the diet program is built to burn the fat for energy.)

To illustrate this point, I have my patients imagine their bloodstream as a banquet table overloaded with sugary foods (this overloaded table represents the A1C of 8.5). As the diner consumes the high-calorie and sugary foods on the table, the quantity of food on the table decreases, but the fat on the diner's body increases. For years I've heard patients lament that their insulin or oral medications make them fat. The truth is that the medication lowered their blood sugar by transferring excess sugar out of the blood and into their fat cells. The insulin didn't make them fat; the excess sugar in the blood (that would have ultimately done long-term damage to the body) moving from the bloodstream into fat cells made them fat. It is vitally important to get excess blood sugar out of the bloodstream and into the fat cells where it can be dieted and exercised away.

It is important to note that the complications from diabetes are typically the result of blood sugar that has been out of control for a long time. Almost all are vascular in nature because long-term exposure of the blood vessels to sticky, syrupy, high concentrations of sugar can cause permanent vessel and nerve damage.

The main areas of diabetes complications are the retina of the eye, kidneys, nerves, heart, brain, gastrointestinal (GI) tract, and dental health, which are all due to vessel or nerve damage from blood sugar that remains out of control.

Arteriosclerosis (Vessel Disease)

Uncontrolled diabetes is associated with earlier and more severe vascular changes than normally occur at a given age. The leading cause of death for those with uncontrolled diabetes is cardiovascular disease.

The incidence of coronary vessel blockage in those with diabetes has been estimated at from 8 to 17 percent. Diabetic adults have heart disease–related deaths and strokes about two times as high as the general population. (Remember that even those with Met B or prediabetes are more prone to midline fat, hypertension, high cholesterol, high triglycerides, and high blood sugar, all setting the stage for heart attacks or strokes.)

Blood vessels that run through the legs to the toes (in the lower extremities) are prone to peripheral vascular disease (PVD). PVD causes disturbed sensation, such as burning, steady pain, intermittent shooting pains on exertion, decrease in muscle endurance, and loss of circulation or pulses in the lower legs and feet. PVD can lead to gangrene and amputation.

Diabetic gangrene usually involves the toes or heels and tends to begin after foot trauma, infection, or extremes in temperature. Because of nerve-related loss of sensation, a person with diabetes may not realize she has a foot infection, cut, or burn that won't heal because she is no longer sensitive to pain in the feet or toes. Careful daily visual inspection of the feet is a good habit to get into for those with diabetes. Take a magnifying mirror and look at the bottom of your feet on a daily basis to catch irritation or cuts as soon as they occur. It is also prudent to remove your socks when you see your doctor for a physical. Remind your physician that you have diabetes and would like your feet inspected and your pulses and circulation checked.

Nephropathy (Kidney Disease)

The kidneys resemble two sacs filled with miles of tiny tubules and blood vessels and are the primary filters of blood in your body. They remove wastes via urine. Years of high-sugar, syrupy blood cause these vessels to harden, become less pliable, crack, and become less able to filter the blood. As a result, high levels of waste products begin to build up in the bloodstream as the kidneys become less able to filter out toxins and release them in the urine. At the same time, some valuable products (such as proteins) are leaked into the urine. The blood contains more waste, and the urine contains more valuable ingredients.

Diabetes is the leading cause of end-stage renal disease in the United States and accounts for about 40 percent of new cases. Nephropathy rarely occurs in the first ten years of diabetes, and it usually takes more than twenty years of uncontrolled blood sugar before kidneys begin to fail. About half the people with diabetes for twenty-plus years have some evidence of renal disease. Less than 10 percent of these people have full-blown nephrotic syndrome with hypertension (high blood pressure), protein in the urine, and edema (swelling).

After years of damage to the kidneys, they can lose so much function that your blood becomes filled with toxins. This is determined by blood and urine tests. If a kidney transplant is not an option, hemodialysis or peritoneal dialysis may be necessary. Both types of dialysis take the place of your kidneys to rid your blood of harmful wastes, extra electrolytes, and water. Hemodialysis uses machinery whereas peritoneal dialysis uses the peritoneal membrane of your stomach to filter your blood.

Retinopathy, Glaucoma, Cataracts (Eye Disease)

It usually takes more than ten years of poorly controlled diabetes for diabetic retinopathy to develop. Some degree of retinopathy is usually present in people who have had diabetes for twenty-plus years. The blood vessels of the retina are very small in diameter.* Years of elevated sugar hardens and crystallizes the tiny veins and capillaries. The damage of retinal disease is often quiet because the retina is located behind the optic nerve. A person may have 20/20 vision but still have damage to the retina. As years pass, advanced stages of retinopathy, termed proliferative retinopathy, cause bleeding, hem-

---

*The diameter of the blood vessels contained in the kidneys is approximately the same diameter as the blood vessels in the retina of the eye. Both the vessels in the retina and in the kidney are naturally very small.

orrhages, retinal detachment, and other serious forms of deterioration. When retinopathy progresses to this late stage, total blindness can occur. (Blindness occurs in only six percent of people with diagnosed retinopathy.) Diabetes is the leading cause of blindness in adults 20 to 74 years of age.

Cataracts and glaucoma are also related to high blood sugar, and both can lead to visual impairment or blindness. There is treatment for diabetes-related eye diseases. The cornerstone to any treatment is returning and keeping blood sugar in the normal range to stop the disease process. Laser therapy can be used to stop the bleeding of retinopathy, medications can be prescribed to lower the pressure in the eye from glaucoma, and surgery is used for cataract removal.

Infections

People with uncontrolled diabetes are prone to infection for several reasons. The natural environment inside the body is dark, warm, and moist. A person with uncontrolled diabetes has a high concentration of blood sugar, providing the perfect food source for bacteria. When infection-causing bacteria take hold, the high sugar environment is perfect for proliferation, making infections stronger and harder to kill in those with diabetes.

Not only will the bacteria thrive in high blood sugar, but sickness naturally causes the release of stress hormones that force blood sugar to rise even higher. High sugar weakens the immune system. People with diabetes are prone to foot infections, yeast infections, urinary tract infections, and surgical site infections. Often a day or two before an infection produces telltale symptoms, a person's blood sugar readings begin to elevate without explanation.

Damage to the blood vessels, nerve damage, and decreased blood flow to the extremities can make it difficult for medications to reach the site of infection and can increase the rate of reinfection or inability to heal.

Because high blood sugar can weaken your immune system, routine vaccinations are very important. Consider getting a yearly flu vaccine, the pneumonia vaccine (if you are age 65 or older, you may need a five-year booster shot), a tetanus shot (with 10-year boosters), and perhaps the hepatitis B vaccine.

Neuropathy (Nerve Damage)

Diabetic neuropathy is the most frequent complication of long-term diabetes. About 65 percent of those with diabetes have mild to severe nervous system damage. Neuropathy's symptoms can run the gamut from chronic aches to shooting pains to burning sensations to lack of sensation or numbness and tingling. Pain is the chief symptom and tends to worsen at night when the person is at rest. It is usually relieved by activity and aggravated by cold. Some people experience cramping, tenderness, and muscle weakness.

Although diabetic neuropathy is the most prevalent complication of type 2 diabetes, it gets the least attention. Most people with diabetes are unaware that the following maladies can be the result of diabetic neuropathy:

- Irregular heartbeat (nerve damage can cause irregular heart rhythm)
- Irregular movement of food/waste down the GI tract (nerve damage can cause gastroparesis with alternating bouts of diarrhea and constipation)
- Excessive or absent perspiration
- Carpal tunnel syndrome
- Urinary and fecal incontinence
- Edema
- Impotence, erectile dysfunction (ED). It is estimated that about 50 percent of diabetic males have some degree of ED.

Of all the complications from uncontrolled diabetes, neuropathies often improve with control of blood sugar. They may not be completely rectified, and it may take several weeks or months to show maximum improvement in symptoms.

Dental Problems

High blood sugar decreases the production of saliva and increases the development of dental plaque. The gums are packed with tiny blood vessels that can become irritated and inflamed from high blood sugar, causing the tissue surrounding the teeth and gums to become prone to infection.

Consider brushing your teeth at least twice a day, floss daily, and schedule dental exams at least twice a year. Consult your dentist if your gums begin to bleed or get red and swollen. Good dental and gum health is essential for good heart health because it appears that the bacteria present in gum disease may trigger blood clots, which can contribute to a heart attack or stroke.

Always remind your dentist and dental hygienist that you have type 2 diabetes so they will be especially vigilant with your cleaning and examination.

Liver Disease

Poorly controlled blood sugar increases the risk for nonalcoholic fatty liver disease (NAFLD). Fat deposits in the liver can lead to scarring of the liver itself (nonalcoholic cirrhosis). The liver is the organ of the body with the most functions, and its optimal health is essential to lead a healthy life. High cholesterol, excess insulin production, insulin resistance, and excessive production of triglycerides can also increase the risk for fatty liver disease. People with Met B, prediabetes, and type 2 diabetes are often prescribed statins to decrease their cholesterol level, but unfortunately, many statins place increased stress and strain on the already compromised liver.

After this discussion of daily and long-term complications of uncontrolled diabetes, and armed with the knowledge of how a healthy body should work, you are now ready to take on the Diabetes Miracle Plan.

PART TWO

THE DIABETES MIRACLE PLAN: REST, RESET, AND RETRAIN THE PANCREAS

INTRODUCTION TO THE DIABETES MIRACLE PLAN

The Diabetes Miracle lifestyle program is designed to put you in control of diabetes. It is a lifestyle rather than a diet. Many people seem to think of diets and dieting as "something I will do to get a better A1C or help me lose a few pounds before I see my doctor." We all want the quick fix that will correct our blood sugar and weight situation immediately, but what we don't take into account is that we will have Met B or diabetes for the rest of our lives and need to learn to decrease weight and be healthy for now and forever.

Unlike many "diets" that only work while you are in a stage of deprivation, the Diabetes Miracle is designed to nonmedicinally correct hormonal imbalance. The goal is not to live in deprivation but rather to live a full life eating the foods you like, in a way that matches your metabolic nature. The Diabetes Miracle is a lifestyle—a very livable and realistic lifestyle—that will get your weight and blood glucose levels into normal range . . . and keep them there. It is scientifically proven, is based on actual physiology, and is designed to match the metabolic needs of the millions of people who truly cannot lose weight; keep it off; and stay healthy on traditional diets, even those written specifically for diabetes. It is the missing link in dieting that will enable you to lose weight and keep it off. Additional benefits include:

Being able to decrease the dosages or number of medications you take—or may even eliminate the need for medications currently used to band-aid any one of the many health conditions that can go hand in hand with elevated blood sugar. Many people with diabetes are on several oral medications or oral medications plus insulin and still do not have normal lab results. The majority of people with diabetes take medications for hypertension, cholesterol, triglycerides, and depression too. The Diabetes Miracle is designed to give you the best chance of needing the least amount of medication with normal blood sugar and improved overall lab work.

Potentially stopping the progression of Metabolism B before it reaches diabetes. For a long time, the progression from Met B to prediabetes to type 2 diabetes was typically exacerbated by recommended high-carb diets as well as medications that forced the pancreas to work harder and fatigue quicker. Most people found themselves progressing from treating their diabetes with diet and exercise to adding pills to maybe even requiring insulin. Now, it's a whole new ball game. Every day, people are slowing or halting the progression of Metabolism B and diabetes.

Decreasing the risk of diabetes complications. These complications can affect nerves, kidneys, heart, vascular system, brain, and circulation . . . in other words, the complications of diabetes affect the entire body. Having diabetes does not mean you will develop complications, but having diabetes out of control does ensure diabetes-related problems. The Diabetes Miracle program quickly normalizes blood sugar and can add healthy years to your lifetime.

Regulating blood sugar to help prevent highs and lows. This regulation helps the body mimic normal metabolism with smooth levels of blood sugar all day and all night, for 24/7 blood sugar control.

Improving the way you feel. It improves energy, focus, concentration, and libido while decreasing fatigue, depression, irritability, carb cravings, and insatiable appetite.

Targeting midline fat. The Diabetes Miracle works to balance insulin release and immediately targets midline fat, muffin top, love handles, and back fat—it is the permanent cure for the apple shape.

Permanent improvement of nutrition-related lab work. These results include total cholesterol, HDL cholesterol, LDL cholesterol, triglycerides, blood sugar, insulin, hemoglobin A1C, and vitamin D levels.

WHAT YOU CAN EXPECT

The Diabetes Miracle is a three-step program that will help you to reset your metabolism by resting your pancreas and liver (Step 1) and reprogramming them to accept and process carbs in a more normal manner (Step 2). You will learn how to control the type, amount, and frequency of the carbs you eat (Step 3). Everything you need to know to live a lifestyle that can help you to become the healthiest person you can be is found within the next chapters. The program is designed specifically to match the metabolic state of a person with Met B, prediabetes, or type 2 diabetes.

The Diabetes Miracle lifestyle decreases the automatic self-feeding mechanism of the liver. You will learn to feed your body the appropriate amount of carbohydrate at the right time to decrease the number of times per day the liver might intervene. As you learn to consume carbohydrates at appropriate intervals and eliminate long gaps without eating, your blood sugar will respond with smooth, normal blood sugar curves.

The program recommends a specified allotment of gentle carbs at designated times, enabling your blood sugar to rise gradually. This smooth blood sugar curve does not force the pancreas to overrelease insulin quickly and urgently. These gentle carbs are considered to be lower in glycemic index and are higher in fiber than high-impact, high–glycemic index carbs. (See box on page 117).

From as early as the fourth day of Step 1, the program will begin to rest your overworking or fatigued pancreas, decrease your liver's workload, and quiet the progressive metabolic mayhem while setting the stage to enable these organs to coexist in a normal metabolic environment. Your blood sugar will begin to dramatically improve after Day 4. In less than a week, you may see major improvement and consistency in blood sugar and free yourself from roller-coaster highs and lows. After Day 4, you will flip on the fat burning switch to shrink the size of fat cells and improve the connection of your own insulin to your cells. Decreased insulin resistance will reduce the stress on the pancreas and allow it to return to producing a normal amount of insulin.

In Step 2, when carbohydrate is added back into the diet, the program is designed like no other. It promotes continued normal blood sugar levels by defining the right type, timing, and amount of carbohydrate to consume throughout the day, at bedtime, and even during the early morning hours to obtain the smooth blood sugar curves that allow for normal insulin release. Eating according to the Diabetes Miracle program generates the amount of blood sugar your body can handle without causing blood sugar levels to roller-coaster and over- or under-insulin release.

Physical activity enables muscle cells to burn blood sugar for fuel, leaving less sugar in the blood that could provoke the pancreas. After an exercise session, empty muscle cells will preferentially flag insulin, decreasing the amount of insulin left to open fat cells. By living a

THE IMPORTANCE OF GLYCEMIC INDEX AND GLYCEMIC LOAD

You've probably heard the recommendation, "Eat more complex carbs and fewer simple carbs." This overly simplistic theory was built on the premise that complex carbs must be healthier than simple carbs. It is a mistake that the more complex in structure a carbohydrate is, the less impact it has on blood sugar and insulin. Avoiding simple carbs, such as jelly beans, and consuming more complex carbs, such as potatoes and pasta, was not the whole story.

The glycemic index is a numerical scale used to indicate how fast and how high a carbohydrate food will raise blood glucose. Carbs are compared to a glycemic index of 100 (assigned to white bread). All the carbohydrate foods are compared equally in portions of 50 grams.

A low–glycemic index food will prompt a slower, more moderate rise in blood sugar, whereas a high glycemic rise will cause a very fast, high spike in blood sugar that can jolt the pancreas into releasing insulin quicker and harder.

Would you believe that the glycemic index of jelly beans and that of a white potato are nearly identical? Both are high–glycemic index foods of about 74–76 on the glycemic index. So avoiding jelly beans while increasing intake of white potatoes would do nothing to help blood sugar. In fact, eating more of certain complex carbs can cause more fat formation on and in the body than some simple carbs.

Glycemic load (GL) takes it one step further in looking at the speed and rise in blood sugar while also taking into account the typical amount of the carbohydrate consumed. For example, you might easily consume 1 cup of pasta but would be unlikely to consume 1 cup of raisins. So, glycemic load involves the impact of carbs in the amount you are apt to consume them.

The Diabetes Miracle program takes into account **both** glycemic index and glycemic load by focusing on a particular quantity of low– to medium–glycemic index foods.

sedentary lifestyle, you are sending the majority of your insulin to your fat cells and setting yourself up to gain fat. Physical activity is a core principle of the Diabetes Miracle.

The program promotes a liberal intake of water or decaffeinated fluid (caffeine is a diuretic and actually promotes dehydration). When a body has the potential to face higher-than-normal blood sugar, it is more prone to dehydration and a higher concentration of toxins and waste products in its blood. Breakdown products from fat burning (called ketones) can lower blood pH and slow fat loss. Adequate hydration rids the body of waste products, toxins, and ketones through the urine.

Diabetes is an inflammatory condition that brings inherent stress to the body. Those with diabetes need to ensure that their intake of stress vitamins (B vitamins) is adequate. Because those with diabetes are more prone to low levels of vitamin D and problems with bone density, including osteoporosis and osteopenia, supplementation with calcium and vitamin D is also recommended. The suggested supplements are added insurance that you are consuming all the nutrients your body requires to maintain health and well-being.

The Diabetes Miracle supports the need for adequate sleep and stress reduction. Stress (whether it is physical or emotional) causes a rise in stress hormones that cause blood sugar to spike. Excessive stress causes diabetes to spiral out of control. The program encourages you to acknowledge, identify, and address stress to create the right environment for optimal blood sugar control. During the sleep cycle, the body (with the help of hormones) repairs and rejuvenates itself for the next day. The Diabetes Miracle encourages you to invest adequate time in sleep to set the day's stage for a healthier blood sugar base.

Within just a few weeks, you will experience much improved blood sugar readings. At the end of the first eight weeks, you will have rested your overworked pancreas and liver, you will have improved the connection of your insulin to insulin receptors, and you will be ready to reprogram the pancreas and liver by presenting them with the correct amount and type of carbohydrate at the right time. The result will be pristine blood sugar on as little medication as possible, continued weight loss, improved cholesterol, triglycerides, blood pressure, and a new lease on a healthy future. Now, that is a miracle!

EIGHT IMPORTANT GUIDELINES

Before you begin the Diabetes Miracle lifestyle, look over the following eight guidelines. It's important that you commit to taking the best care of yourself if your body is to improve in health and energy. These guidelines are the backbone of the program and will support you during your transformation to great blood sugar, improved health, and bountiful energy.

GUIDELINE 1

Follow the roadmap of *The Diabetes Miracle* to get to your final destination: normal blood sugar, increased energy, improved health, and desired weight.

The Diabetes Miracle is a lifetime program that consists of three steps. Because you begin the program with a metabolism that is out of control, you have to start at the beginning and follow the steps in order. Jumping in at Step 2 will not rest your pancreas or liver, and you will not reap the benefits of the program.

Step 1: Rehab, Detox, Boot camp. This initial step lasts a minimum of eight weeks, but you can remain in Step 1 longer if you choose. These eight weeks will rest the overworking pancreas/liver combination, almost immediately improve your blood sugar readings, put the body into a fat burning mode (burning body fat as well as decreasing cholesterol and triglycerides), and decrease insulin release and insulin resistance.

During Step 1, you will be eating a lower-carbohydrate diet, but it is certainly not carb-free. Step 1 is a short-term, low-carb step that is a means to an end. Although powerful carbs that have a high glycemic index (such as pasta, rice, cereal, and fruit) are eliminated for these eight weeks, many foods that contain marginal amounts of carbohydrate are considered neutral and can be eaten freely in addition to the recommended liberal intake of lean protein, heart-healthy fat, and neutral veggies. To top it off, you have the option of adding a 5 gram "counter" carb to each meal and bedtime snack, allowing the inclusion of low-carb versions of bread, wraps, yogurt, crackers, desserts, and treats.

Step 2: Transition or Reprogramming. The second step begins immediately after first and lasts a minimum of eight weeks or until you reach your desired weight or size, and your lab work is in the normal range with little to no medication. Everything that was legal in Step 1 remains legal in Step 2, and you will begin to reintroduce low-impact carbs in the right amount at the right time to allow for continued blood sugar control, weight loss, energy, and improved health.

You will notice that Step 2 resembles a normal way of eating with carbohydrate, protein, fat, and veggies in balanced meals. The way you eat in Step 2 will become the backbone for Step 3.

Step 3: A Lifestyle, Not a Diet. At this stage, you will have an increased amount and variety of carbohydrates as well as lean protein, heart-healthy fat, and neutral veggies to provide a balanced, nutritious, and very livable lifestyle. This lifestyle aims to maintain normal blood sugar, your desired weight, and healthy lab work for a lifetime. Balance is the key.

Guideline 2

Hydration: Everyone with prediabetes or type 2 diabetes experiences higher-than-normal blood sugar that results in a higher-than-normal daily requirement for water or decaf fluid. Dehydration puts greater strain on the kidneys and can result in changes in blood pH and concentration of minerals and waste products. Steps 1 and 2 are fat-burning stages that create waste products from fat's breakdown. When dehydration occurs, ketones (the waste products produced from burning fat) build in the blood, changing its pH to become slightly more acidic. The brain detects this change in pH and purposely slows fat-burning in an effort to help neutralize the blood. Add to that an increased concentration of blood sugar, and you can see the importance of drinking water. Drinking water will help you to lose more fat and keep your blood at its proper concentration. Over the course of each day, you should strive to drink a minimum of 64 ounces of water or decaffeinated fluid. (People 5 feet 3 inches or less should drink a minimum of 48 ounces). Increase fluid intake when you exercise: Consider adding 8 ounces of water for every fifteen minutes of exercise on a hot day. You may either spread your fluid intake throughout the day or drink more in the morning and less in the evening. Although coffee, tea, and caffeine-containing sugar-free beverages are allowed on all steps of the program, don't count them in your 64 ounce fluid intake because caffeine is a diuretic and actually promotes dehydration.

GUIDELINE 3

Eat Throughout the Day: The old-school diabetes diet was three meals and a bedtime snack. The Diabetes Miracle lifestyle requires that you eat throughout the day (and even into the night if you are awake). In Step 1, you will learn that many food choices are neutral and have no major impact on blood sugar, insulin, or excess fat accumulation. Neutral foods can be eaten liberally at any time. Unnaturally restricting your intake of neutral foods will not speed fat burning. When you feel hungry on Step 1, eat—but make sure you are choosing neutral foods.

The Diabetes Miracle diet is set up like bookends: You should eat your first meal or snack within one hour of waking and eat a snack within one hour of going to sleep at night. Don't allow more than five hours to pass during the day without eating. If you are awake in the middle of the night, you can eat an appropriate snack as well. The mind-set is: Start the day eating, end the night eating. If you are awake in the middle of the night, you may eat, and if the time between any meals exceeds five hours, make sure to snack between the meals.

Although most calorie-based diets strongly caution to stop eating after 6:00 or 7:00 PM, it is now known that whenever more than five hours pass without eating, the liver will automatically and naturally release glycogen stores. In the case of a person with prediabetes or type 2 diabetes, this survival amount of glycogen will cause blood sugar to rise higher than if the person ate a snack prior to the liver release.

Jay ate breakfast at 8:00 AM and lunch at 1:30 PM, so as far as he was concerned, he had eaten two meals. What Jay did not know was that at about 1:00 PM, his liver released sugar in an automatic response. If he had checked his blood sugar before eating lunch (at the five and a half hour mark since breakfast), he might have been shocked to see an increase in his blood sugar.

To prevent the liver from unnecessary behind-the-scenes overfeeding, you must eat. When you wake up, your first meal or snack stops the liver from dispensing sugar stores. When you have a snack right before bedtime, you will buy five hours into the night without liver interference. Blocking excess liver release of sugar is an important aspect of controlling blood sugar and insulin release. Spreading food out over a twenty-four-hour period puts you in control of your blood sugar all day and all night.

GUIDELINE 4

Exercise: For those who are not regular exercisers, you needn't join a gym or get a personal trainer to live the Diabetes Miracle lifestyle. However, you do need to increase your physical activity over and above your normal activity by a minimum of thirty minutes, five times per week. This exercise doesn't need to be done all at once, but by the end of most days, you should have added a minimum of thirty minutes to your typical daily activity. One form of exercise isn't better than another; in fact, a variety of physical activities is better than doing the same exercise for the same length of time at the same time of day. Choose activities that you enjoy, and do one on one day, another on another. Walk, ride your bike, go for a swim, work in the garden, take a yoga class, or work out at the gym—whatever you'd like. If you are wheelchair bound or are unsteady on your feet, armchair exercise is just fine. Any type of movement that gets your muscles working is the key.

EXERCISE AND MUSCLE MOVEMENT LOWERS BLOOD SUGAR LEVELS IN THREE WAYS:

First, active muscle cells consume blood sugar for fuel. Envision your muscles as mini-furnaces that extract sugar from the blood both during and for hours after your actual exercise session is over. If you do not exercise, your inactive muscle cells would have no need to consume blood sugar for activity, and your blood sugar would remain higher than if you had exercised.

Second, muscle cells contain their own stores of glycogen (stored sugar). When you begin to exercise, these stores are mobilized. When you eat a meal or snack after having exercised, the emptied muscle cells will flag insulin to open receptors and allow them to refill with sugar. This is another way exercise helps decrease sugar in the blood.

Third, exercise can help lower blood sugar can be described by imagining the concept of *red* cells (active muscle cells) versus *blue* cells (inactive fat cells or unexercised muscle cells). Use the color analogy to describe the concept that exercised muscle cells become metabolically active and might appear to the brain as red, whereas metabolically inactive fat cells or unexercised muscles cells could appear blue. When the brain is deciding where to acquire fuel while you are on a fat-burning diet, it will spare the red muscle cells, noting that they are functioning and active and will preferentially choose to consume the blue inactive cells. If you don't exercise, both inactive muscle and fat cells appear blue, and the brain will choose to consume some muscle as well as some fat for energy. Exercising while living the Diabetes Miracle lifestyle spares your muscles and puts you in a 100 percent fat-burning mode.

---

*See Chapter 12 for more on exercise.

When it comes to stress, those with prediabetes or type 2 diabetes must focus on keeping their life as calm as possible. Exercise can help to combat the release of stress hormones that normally cause blood sugar to rise. Increasing movement on a stressful day will lower your blood sugar and decrease your chance for needing increased medication or gaining excess stress-related weight.

Unlike standard exercise recommendations that suggest warming up for five to ten minutes, followed by a minimum of thirty minutes of aerobic-type exercise, and then five to ten minutes of a cool down, people with type 2 diabetes and Met B actually benefit more from spreading their exercise throughout the day. For example: You may choose to do forty minutes of walking after breakfast in the morning, and that would fulfill your physical activity requirement for the day. This would empty glycogen from muscle cells, attract insulin to refill muscle cells, increase metabolism, and help decrease blood sugar for hours afterward. However, you might get a greater benefit by splitting your activity into two twenty-minute sessions—twenty minutes of walking after breakfast and twenty minutes of walking after dinner. This will fulfill your physical activity requirement for the day, empty glycogen from muscle cells twice a day, attract insulin twice a day, and increase metabolism for hours after both meals. You are doing the same amount of exercise with a bigger bang.

No matter how you choose to do it, the idea is to move your muscles over and above your typical activity level for a minimum of thirty minutes a day, five days a week.

Guideline 5

Take Vitamins, Minerals, and Supplements: Vitamins, minerals, and supplements can provide the extra insurance that you will meet your daily vitamin and mineral requirements. They are particularly helpful during the most restrictive Step 1 but can and should be taken during all the steps of the Diabetes Miracle. Always check with your physician before taking supplements, and consider adding them to the medication list you keep in your wallet with your identification.

It's often easier to remember to take supplements with a meal, and many of them will absorb more readily if you do so. Take your vitamins right after you eat your meal. I recommend taking them at two different sessions as follows.

To take right after breakfast or lunch:

Multivitamin with minerals

Fish oil (suggested 1000–1200 mg)

Calcium with vitamin D (suggested 500–600 mg calcium with
approximately 200 IU vitamin D3)

Extra vitamin D supplement if indicated (if physician agrees, you
may require an additional 1000 IU vitamin D3 a day based on
your vitamin D level).

To take following dinner:

B-complex (suggested B-50)

Fish oil (suggested 1000–1200 mg)

Calcium with vitamin D (suggested 500–600 mg plus 200 IU
vitamin D3)

Vitamin E (400 IU) with doctor approval.

Multivitamin/Mineral Supplement. There are many excellent multivitamin/mineral supplements available. Many multivitamins are targeted to your specific age and gender. Step 1 is a short-term phase that is necessary to rest the pancreas and liver, but it requires that all powerful carbs are eliminated for eight weeks. These carb foods normally provide fiber, antioxidants, minerals, and vitamins. They will be reintroduced to your diet after eight weeks, but in the meantime, you should consider taking the suggested multivitamins/minerals. Women of childbearing age should consider a supplement that contains iron, while menopausal women and men do not require added iron in their vitamins.

Calcium with Vitamin D. The recommendation is 600 mg of calcium with 200 mg of Vitamin D3 twice a day. Calcium should be taken in two doses because the body can only absorb a maximum of 600 mg at a time. People with Met B, prediabetes, and diabetes have an increased tendency to develop osteopenia (low bone mineral density) and osteoporosis (thinning of bones with progressive bone loss associated with an increased risk of fractures). Recent studies have shown that many are vitamin D deficient. (It appears that imbalance of insulin leads to deficiency of vitamin D.)

Additional vitamin D if you are deficient. Because many people with prediabetes and type 2 diabetes have vitamin D deficiencies, it is wise to have your vitamin D level checked annually to ascertain if an additional supplement is necessary. Remember that you will be getting vitamin D in your multivitamin as well as with your calcium supplement.

If your vitamin D level is under 32, your physician may advise that you take an additional 1000 IU of vitamin D3. As your Met B, prediabetes, or type 2 diabetes regulates, your vitamin D level should hold steady, and the additional supplement might be discontinued based on improvements in your lab work.

Fish Oil. Fish oil has tremendous anti-inflammatory properties. It is also known to fight cancer and heart disease, can lower cholesterol and seems to help with joint mobility. I recommend 2000–2400 mg/day. Make sure that the fish oil supplement you purchase contains a minimum of 60 percent omega 3—every 1000 mg of fish oil should contain at least 600 mg of omega 3. Also, look for fish oil labeled "mercury free." Some cardiologists recommend 4000 mg/day for patients with high cholesterol and inflammatory disease. Fish oil is an excellent source of omega 3 fatty acids DHA and EPA that can help decrease triglycerides, blood pressure, and plaque growth. It also helps act as a blood thinner. (If you take a blood thinner, such as warfarin or Coumadin, check with your doctor before using a fish oil supplement.)

B-complex. B-complex is a combination of eight B vitamins, all of which must be replenished on a daily basis because they are not stored. They can help prevent anemia; increase the rate of metabolism; maintain healthy skin, hair, nerves, and muscle; enhance the immune system; and help balance blood sugar.

Prediabetes and type 2 diabetes are stressful and inflammatory metabolic conditions. By virtue of having blood sugar aberrations, you burn more B vitamins than the average person. B vitamins are water soluble, and excesses leave the body in the urine. I recommend a B-complex (B-50) be taken during one meal; take your multivitamin at another. If you take a multivitamin that is high in B vitamins and take a B-complex at the same time, you are bound to lose the B-complex in your urine.

Vitamin E. Ask your physician about vitamin E supplementation because some physicians prefer to solely use the omega 3 fatty acids of fish oil without additional vitamin E. If he agrees that a supplement would be in your best interest, look for d-alpha tocopherol. Vitamin E has been linked to decreasing coronary vascular disease and may prevent damage to cell membranes from free radicals that can lead to certain types of cancer and inflammation. If you do supplement with E, check the amount of vitamin E in your multivitamin because it contributes to your 400 IU/day.

GUIDELINE 6
Drink Green Tea: Green tea contains a powerful antioxidant, epigallocatechin gallate (EGCG), that has been linked to lowering LDL "bad" cholesterol; improving the HDL:LDL ratio; decreasing the growth of breast, prostate, colon, and skin cancer; and aiding in

midline fat burn. Green tea seems to help decrease constipation and helps to regulate bowel movements. I recommend using a minimum of two tea bags a day. (You can put them in one cup.) Green tea has about half the caffeine of black tea. Make sure to steep your green tea for at least three minutes to obtain the antioxidant potential.

Many companies are capitalizing on the wonderful benefits of steeped green tea leaves by claiming that their capsules, beverages, drops, tablets, and chewing gums contain EGCG. These products might contain the antioxidant but are not the same as drinking green tea steeped from tea leaves. Remember that the antioxidant in green tea is most effective within a few hours of steeping, so make sure to consume it the same day you brew it. Regular green tea contains more EGCG than decaffeinated green tea.*

GUIDELINE 7

Reduce Stress and Think Positive: I am a firm believer that your thoughts and state of mind affect the outcome of your day. If you wake up and think, "Ugh, I am tired, and I don't want to go to that stressful job of mine," you will soon find yourself arriving at work feeling anxious and defeated. Sometimes we are our own worst enemy.

Instead of lamenting, "I have diabetes, just like my mother and her mother. I'm going to be overweight, will eventually need to inject insulin, and will most likely have many health problems as I get older . . . what's the point?" try thinking, "I inherited the gene for diabetes from my mom and her mom. Thankfully, I am diagnosed at a time when diabetes is much better understood. Unlike my mom, I will be able to lose weight and keep it off and may actually be able to control my diabetes with little or no medication. Health problems from diabetes? I don't think so!"

---

*If you are taking a blood thinner (such as warfarin), check with your physician before adding green tea to your daily intake.

STRESS EATING?

Have you ever noticed that some people can't eat a thing when they are stressed, but others can't stop eating? I am willing to bet that those who can't eat during stress have textbook metabolism. Because stress hormones make blood sugar rise, those with Met B, prediabetes, and type 2 diabetes will respond with insulin issues and an insatiable appetite for carbs. Those with uncontrolled Met B often gain weight during stress, while those with Metabolism A usually lose weight.

For a few minutes in the morning before jumping out of bed, and last thing in the evening before falling asleep, take some time to think good thoughts, framing the day in a positive light. Speak to yourself in a positive, kind, motivating, supportive way—you will react in much the same way you would if an outside person was supportive, kind, and motivating.

Get in the habit of taking a few short minutes to relax during the day. Practice deep breathing, visualize peaceful scenes, and think pleasing thoughts. Close your eyes, breathe deeply in and out, and allow your head to clear. A few minutes of deep breathing with your eyes closed and mind clear will help reduce your stress level, blood pressure, blood sugar, and weight.

When it comes to stress, keep in mind that it has a tremendous impact on raising blood sugar. If you are following your meal plan, exercising, drinking adequate water, and so on but experience a highly stressful day, your blood sugar will spike simply because of stress hormones.

GUIDELINE 8

Test Your Blood Sugar, Keep Records, and Show Them to Your Physician: It is close to impossible to know, without testing, if your blood sugar is in or out of normal range. Blood sugar that is significantly elevated (readings over 200 mg/dL) or low blood sugar (readings under 70 mg/dL) may come with symptoms, but moderately high blood sugar may happen without any physical signs or symptoms. Blood sugar out of normal range for an extended period of time will, over time, damage the body. Elevations in blood sugar don't have to be sky-high to cause complications, such as wear and tear on the heart, blood vessels, nerves, retina, and kidneys.

Most people who control their blood sugar with diet and exercise or diet/exercise and oral medication will test their blood sugar twice a day: first thing in the morning upon rising (I aim for 70–120 mg/dL) and two hours after the start of varying meals (I aim for 140 mg/dL or less).

If you take insulin for blood sugar control, most physicians recommend testing pre-meal and at bedtime plus anytime you feel you may have a very high or low reading. The goal of pre-meal readings is usually 80–110 mg/dL, but your physician can help you set your individual goals for pre-meal or bedtime blood sugar.

Keep records of your blood sugar (handwritten in a log book, in the meter's memory, or in a computer printout of a log book), and always bring your readings to your medical appointments. Hand them to your physician and make certain they are addressed. Your lab report only shows your fasting glucose at that one moment in time or a three-month average reading (your hemoglobin A1C is the average of high and low readings during the previous three months).

The readings you obtain from your home monitoring of blood sugar show how your body reacts to the sugar your liver releases during the night (fasting reading) and how you react to the food you have eaten (two hours after the start of a meal reading). Home monitoring can also show your reaction to certain foods, stress, exercise, illness, pain, excess medication, and inadequate medication. Home monitoring gives priceless information that can never be captured during one blood draw at the lab.

STEP 1:
STOPPING THE DIABETES TRAIN

WHAT TO EXPECT IN STEP 1

- **How long is Step 1?** A minimum of eight weeks. (You may remain in Step 1 longer, if desired.)

- **What is the purpose of Step 1?** To temporarily eliminate foods that cause blood sugar to rise and allow the liver to release its glycogen stores. Without significant carbohydrate intake and freed from the liver's deposits of glycogen, blood sugar should normalize within the first week. This new-found equilibrium allows the pancreas and liver to rest.

    For those with prediabetes, Step 1 will calm your overworking pancreas/ liver combination and dramatically decrease the release of the fat-gain hormone insulin. This enables the body to switch to a "fat-burning" mode at the same time Step 1 is normalizing your blood sugar. If you have type 2 diabetes, Step 1 will help to minimize blood sugar spikes and quickly normalize blood sugar so you require less medication. Step 1 will prevent the pancreas from further wear and tear. It also allows for fat-burning both on the body and in the blood. Step 1 stops the blood sugar–based complications of diabetes in their tracks.

    Typically, after approximately four days of Step 1, the body shifts from running on blood sugar produced from both carbs and liver glycogen to burning fat. Fat-burning occurs both in the blood (decreasing LDL cholesterol and triglycerides) and on the body (especially midline fat). However, if you begin Step 1 with very elevated blood fat or blood sugar, it will take more than four days for the body to shift to fat-burning mode.

(Continues)

(Continued)

If you have diabetes, you will not see marked improvement in blood sugar during the first four days of Step 1 because during these days, the liver is releasing stores of glycogen every five hours. After Day 4, you can expect to see blood sugar improvement. If you are taking prescription medications for diabetes, Step 1's quick effect may allow a decrease in medications (with your doctor's approval, of course).

- **How will you feel on Step 1?** During the first few days, you can expect to feel tired, hungry, and irritable and to experience cravings for carbohydrates. However, these feelings will subside. The reason for these symptoms is that your liver is releasing glycogen stores around the clock for four days. Those with prediabetes will typically begin to feel improvement after Day 4 of the program. From Day 4 on, you should feel an uptick in energy, improved mood, no carb cravings, and a decrease in hunger.

If you began the Diabetes Miracle with an HbA1C over 7.0, it may take longer for you to feel the surge in energy because there is excessive sugar in your blood that will need to be assimilated. No matter where you are when you begin, within a matter of days you will be feeling much better, and blood sugar will show marked improvement.

If you're like most people with prediabetes or type 2 diabetes, you are beginning the Diabetes Miracle with an overworked metabolism. Your blood sugar has been roller-coastering for years, and your emotional, physical, psychological health is impaired. Prediabetes means your pancreas is in overdrive making insulin: You have excess insulin in your blood, but insulin resistance on the part of your cells is negating insulin's effectiveness. If you have advanced to type 2 diabetes, the metabolic situation is even more extreme. In either case, your pancreas and liver need a rest—and the sooner, the better.

No matter what your weight or weight-loss goals—if you are 10 pounds or 210 pounds overweight—you will need to remain in Step 1 for a minimum of eight weeks. This program is scientifically based and must be followed as directed to obtain results. The steps are numbered 1, 2, and 3 and must be followed in sequential order to internally rest and rehabilitate your liver and pancreas to allow for more normal metabolism of carbs and glycogen in the future.

Step 1 will put the brakes on your hyperactive or overworked pancreas. Imagine a runaway train rushing down the tracks at 90 miles per hour. When the engineer slams on the brakes, the train won't immediately stop on a dime. The train will gradually slow to a stop. When you begin the Diabetes Miracle, your metabolism is like that runaway train building speed and in danger of derailing. It will take a minimum of four days to get your liver to empty glycogen stores and your pancreas to slow down its insulin response. If you begin the program with very high blood sugar, cholesterol, triglycerides, or insulin levels, it may take longer. Just know that the first days of the Diabetes Miracle are necessary to get your body into fat-burning mode.

If you have diabetes and test your blood sugar, you will probably notice that for the first four days, your blood sugar readings will not show much improvement. The combination of excess sugar in your blood from your previously uncontrolled diabetes and the release of glycogen stores from the liver will make your blood sugar readings erratic. If you have diabetes, don't expect to see any significant improvement in blood sugar until after Day 4.

WHERE YOU BEGIN

People with type 2 diabetes begin the Diabetes Miracle in all different states of control. Remember that HbA1C reflects your average blood sugar for the three months prior to the blood draw. Normal A1C is under 5.7. If you begin the program with an A1C of 6.5, it may take only four days to right the blood sugar in your system and begin the fat-burning. But if you begin Step 1 with an HbA1C of 10.00, it means that your blood sugar on a daily basis is averaging approximately 240 mg/dL. It will certainly take longer than four days to "consume" the excess blood sugar, assimilate it as fat, and begin to burn your body's fat stores. So, the more out of control your blood sugar, the longer it will take you to become symptom-free and regain normal blood sugar on Step 1.

A FAT-BURNING PROGRAM

On the Diabetes Miracle plan, hemoglobin A1C will absolutely correct itself (and with less or no medication if you began the program taking blood sugar medication). I have found that most clinicians don't realize and therefore don't inform their patients that for every point HbA1C drops (improves), about five pounds of fat tissue will form.

For example, if your A1C drops from 7.2 to 6.2, you will have assimilated five pounds of fat as a result of moving that excess blood sugar from the bloodstream into fat cells. Thank goodness that the Diabetes Miracle is a fat-burning program. As quickly as your blood sugar improves and you assimilate that extra fat tissue, the program will burn it off. As a result, you won't gain weight as your blood sugar initially regulates.

An excellent way to burn blood sugar without causing it to be stuffed into fat cells is to exercise. Exercise will allow the muscle cells to consume the excess blood sugar for energy and attract insulin to open and refill your muscles with sugar during the day. So, a combination of Step 1 of the Diabetes Miracle and thirty minutes of increased physical activity five times a week will not cause fat gain as your HbA1C improves. Expect good things: normal blood sugar, a program that will burn the excess fat tissue formed by normalizing sugar, and a whole new you on the other side.

Step 1 is designed to keep your pancreas at rest. If the pancreas and liver reengage, your blood sugar, insulin, and weight will go out of whack again. There is one simple way to accomplish this blood sugar equilibrium: Liberally consume foods that do not convert in any significant way to blood sugar and temporarily avoid foods that raise blood sugar.

SIMPLE RULES FOR STEP 1

1. Eat within one hour of awakening, within one hour of going to bed, and go no longer than five hours without eating. If the time between your meals will exceed five hours, make sure to snack on neu-

tral foods between those meals. If you are awake in the middle of the night, you may certainly snack.

2. You have the option of using a 5 gram counter carb with your neutral foods at breakfast, lunch, dinner, bedtime, and in the middle of the night if you are awake.

3. Drink a minimum of 64 ounces of water or decaffeinated fluid. (If you are 5' 3" or less, drink a minimum 48 ounces of water per day.)

4. Take vitamins, minerals, and other supplements (see page 124 for a list of supplements).

5. Drink green tea using a minimum of two tea bags a day.

6. Exercise a minimum of thirty minutes, five times per week, above your normal activity. Change it up for variety.

STEP 1 FOODS

What to eat. Lean protein, heart-healthy fat, neutral veggies, and limited foods containing 5 grams or less net carbs (5 gram counter carbs).

What to avoid. High-impact carbs must be temporarily avoided (they will be back in Step 2).

Every food on Earth contains nutrients that fit into one or more of three major categories: carbohydrate, protein, or fat. Foods are categorized by the nutrient that is in the greatest supply. Although low-fat milk contains carb, protein, and fat, its nutrient in greatest supply is carbohydrate. As a result, milk is classified as carbohydrate. Likewise, cheese is made of protein and fat, and its protein content classifies it as protein. Butter, which is primarily fat, is classified as fat. On The Diabetes Miracle plan, milk is to be avoided during Step 1, but cheese and butter are neutral. This is because milk will cause blood sugar to rise and engage the pancreas, but cheese and butter will not cause metabolic mayhem.

If during Step 1 you make a mistake and consume an impact carbohydrate, your blood sugar will immediately rise, your liver and muscles will replete with glycogen, your pancreas will engage, and your carb cravings will return. Any impact carbohydrates consumed in a five-hour period sets Step 1 back three days, erasing all the work you did. Resolve to avoid the listed impact carb choices for eight weeks to get the full benefit of Step 1. If you realize you made a mistake in a five-hour block of time, you must add three days to the end of the eight weeks. During the three days after a slip-up, you will feel tired, cranky, and crave carbs again.

NEUTRAL FOODS

Examples of food choices that don't rock the boat on Step 1:

- Protein foods: meat, poultry, fish, soy, nut butters, eggs, cheese
- Fat foods: butter, oil, cream, nuts, seeds, salad dressing, avocado, olives
- Neutral vegetables: broccoli, spinach, lettuce, sprouts, cauliflower, cucumbers, brussels sprouts, artichokes, mushrooms, onions, and peppers. These vegetables are high in vitamins, minerals and fiber, but do not contain significant carbohydrate.

You should familiarize yourself with the Arrow Sheet on pages 138–139 for the many foods that fit into Step 1 and those that are to be temporarily avoided. Many people keep a copy of this arrow sheet on their refrigerator, in their purse, or take it with them as they shop for food. There are many, many neutral choices.

It is critical in Step 1 to temporarily eliminate the foods that spike blood sugar and insulin. For years, people thought that because those with diabetes had high blood sugar, they would have to avoid sugar to achieve good blood sugar levels. However, every single carbohydrate breaks down into blood sugar, not only the sweet carb choices. Although fruit, potatoes, lentils, whole grains, rice, milk, and yogurt are healthy and are loaded with vitamins, minerals, and fiber, their carbohydrate content contributes to your blood sugar, weight, pancreas fatigue, and health woes.

Do not worry—carbs won't be off your plate forever. You will only need to eliminate high-impact or dense carbs for eight weeks. On Step 2, you'll consume healthy carbohydrates in controlled amounts and at proper times to allow for normal blood sugar. In this way, you will program your metabolism to handle carbohydrate foods normally.

If you were to start the Diabetes Miracle at Step 2, skipping the eight weeks of Step 1, you would never succeed at getting your best blood sugar, losing weight, improving LDL and triglycerides, or feeling a tremendous improvement in your symptoms. Step 1 is designed to clean out all the excess blood sugar, burn fats, rest the pancreas, and let your body start Step 2 fresh. Once you are ready for Step 2, you will methodically increase your carb intake in a specific way to allow your body to function more normally.

NEUTRAL PROTEINS (ARROW UP)

Net carb grams is a calculation that measures total carbs minus fiber grams in a certain quantity of food. More on that later when you will learn to determine net carbs of the 5 gram counter foods you may choose to eat in Step 1 (see page 144 for formula).

There is no need to check Nutrition Facts for net carb grams for the following foods:
- Poultry: skinless chicken and turkey, Cornish game hen, lean ground turkey, lean ground chicken, turkey bacon (nitrite- or nitrate-free recommended)
- Lean beef: filet, flank steak, sirloin, T-Bone trimmed, ground round, Porterhouse trimmed, steak, London broil, 85–93 percent ground beef, tenderloin, rib roast, rump roast, round chuck roast
- Fish and shellfish: poached, broiled, baked, sautéed (NO breading)

THE
Arrow Sheet

YES
For all steps

PROTEIN ARROW
(Lean, lite, or low-fat preferred)

Meat
Poultry
Fish and shellfish
Cheese
Cottage cheese
Eggs
Egg substitutes

Natural nut butter
Natural seed butter
Tofu
Unsweetened soy milk
Edamame
*Select protein shakes

Although meats and cheeses are primarily protein, they vary tremendously in their fat content. The recommended protein sources in the Diabetes Miracle program will be heart healthy and lean. You can feel free to enjoy them liberally.

YES
For all steps

FAT ARROW
(Lite or low-fat preferred)

Butter
Margarine
Sour cream
Mayonnaise
Cream
Half-and-half

Oil
Salad dressing
Olives
Avocados
Nuts
Seeds
Whipped Cream

YES
For all steps

NEUTRAL VEGGIES ARROW

Artichokes and artichoke hearts
Asparagus
Green or wax beans
Bean sprouts
Broccoli
Brussels sprouts
Cabbage
Cauliflower

Celery
Cucumbers
Dill Pickles
Eggplant
Jicama (max 1 cup)
Onions and scallions
Greens (collards, kale, mustard, turnip, spinach)

Kohlrabi
Leeks
Mushrooms
Okra
Peppers (all varieties)
Lettuce and other salad greens
Radishes
Spaghetti squash

Sauerkraut
Tomatoes (maximum 1 fresh tomato per meal or 10 cherry tomatoes, ½ cup canned tomatoes, ½ cup tomato salsa, ½ cup tomato sauce (no sugar), ½ cup tomato or veggie juice
Turnips
Zucchini and summer squash

Bread
Wraps
Rolls
Buns
Bread Products
Pasta
Rice

Crackers, pretzels, chips
Cereal and granola bars
Cereal (hot or cold)
Other grains
Fruit
Fruit juice
Potatoes and sweet potatoes

CARBOHYDRATE ARROW
(Carbohydrate foods will require label check for Steps 1 and 3)

Carrots
Parsnips
Beets
Winter squash
Acorn squash
Pumpkin
Milk

Yogurt
Sweetened beverages
Sweets and desserts
Carb-containing foods that fail the 5 gram "counter" test

NO for Step 1

YES for all Steps
*5 GRAM "COUNTER" CARBS
(Step 1: optional at meals and bedtime snacks. Steps 2 and 3: can be added into carb total for a meal/snack on Steps 2 and 3.)

*Low-carb bread
*Low-carb tortillas
*Low-carb wraps
*Low-carb crackers
*Low-carb yogurts

*Low-carb juices
*Low-carb milk
*Low-carb protein drinks with 2–5 grams net carb
*Foods or recipes in the serving size that provide 5 or less grams net carb

*All of the starred foods must pass the net carb test and fit the 5 gram "counter" carb rule (page 41).
Net carb grams 1 gram = neutral

- Pork: pork tenderloin, ham, Canadian bacon, trimmed pork chops
- Lamb: roast lamb, lamb chop, leg of lamb
- Veal: lean veal chop, veal roast
- Game: venison, skinless duck and pheasant, ostrich, buffalo, rabbit, deer
- Cheese: cottage cheese, ricotta, string cheese, mozzarella, grated cheese (low-fat preferred)
- Eggs: whole eggs, egg whites, egg substitute
- Soy and soy products: tofu, unsweetened and unflavored soy milk, vegetarian meat substitutes (without added carbohydrates)
- Natural nut and seed butters (containing nuts or seeds, oil, or salt): almond butter, cashew butter, tahini.

NEUTRAL FATS (ARROW UP)

There is no need to check nutrition facts for net carb grams for the following foods:

- Butter: light or low-fat preferred, whipped, butter blends (one-half butter, one-half oil)
- Margarine: light or low-fat preferred, tub, whipped
- Sour cream and cream cheese: light or low-fat preferred, whipped
- Cream or half-and-half: light or low-fat preferred, light whipped cream
- Oils: olive, canola, peanut, corn, safflower, sunflower, soybean
- Salad Dressing: vinaigrette, light or low-fat preferred (avoid fat free)
- Mayonnaise: light or low-fat preferred
- Olives
- Avocado

- Nuts: almonds, peanuts, cashews, walnuts, pecans, macadamia nuts, pistachios (avoid coatings, such as honey or cinnamon sugar, that contain carbohydrate)
- Seeds: sesame seeds, sunflower seeds, pumpkin seeds, tahini paste (sesame seed paste).

NEUTRAL VEGETABLES (ARROW UP)

There is no need to check nutrition facts for net carb grams for the following foods:

- Artichoke and hearts
- Asparagus
- Bean sprouts
- Beans (green and wax)
- Broccoli
- Brussels sprouts
- Cabbage
- Cauliflower
- Celery
- Cucumber
- Dill pickles
- Eggplant
- Greens (mustard, turnip, collards, kale, spinach)
- Kohlrabi
- Leeks
- Lettuces and salad greens
- Mushrooms
- Okra
- Onions/scallions
- Peppers
- Radishes
- Rutabaga
- Spaghetti squash

- Sauerkraut
- Tomatoes (one per meal)
    — Cherry tomatoes (ten per meal)
    — Crushed or canned tomatoes (one-half cup per meal)
- Tomato salsa (one-half cup per meal)
- Tomato and vegetable juices (maximum 4 ounces per meal)
- Marinara sauce, containing tomatoes and seasonings only–(one-half cup per meal maximum)
- Turnips
- Zucchini and summer squash.

FREEBIES ON STEP 1

During Step 1, you can eat these foods whenever you like because they contain negligible carbohydrate grams (net carb grams of 1 gram or less):

- Sugar-free gelatin
- Sugar-free chewing gum
- Zero-carb jelly
- Zero-carb syrup
- Bouillon
- Broth
- Consommé
- Club soda
- Diet soda
- Sugar-free tonic
- Select fitness water, flavored waters, and flavored seltzers
- Coffee, tea
- White horseradish
- Lemon and lime juice
- Mustard
- Dill pickles
- Vinegar
- All herbs and spices
- Salad dressing sprays
- Soy sauce.

STEP 1 CARBS TO AVOID—HIGH-IMPACT CARBS (ARROW DOWN)

- Breads: bread, wraps, pitas, bagels, waffles, pancakes, muffins, croissants, and rolls
- Pasta: white, semolina, and whole-grain
- Rice: wild, white, basmati, or brown rice
- Crackers, pretzels, and chips with 5 grams or more net carbs
- Protein bars and snack bars with 5 grams or more net carbs
- Cereal and grains: oatmeal, barley, grits, and dry breakfast cereals
- Fruit or fruit juice
- Sweetened drinks: soda, teas, punch, and energy drinks
- Certain vegetables: carrots; parsnips; winter squash; acorn squash; pumpkin; beets; legumes or dried beans, such as lentils, black beans, limas, kidney beans, or cannelloni beans; peas; potatoes, including white potatoes and sweet potatoes; quinoa
- Sweets and desserts
- Milk: skim, 1 percent, 2 percent, and buttermilk
- Yogurt with 5 grams or more net carbs: yogurt, low-calorie yogurt, regular yogurt
- Sweetened, flavored soy milk.

FIVE GRAM CARB COUNTERS

These are optional treats that you can have at breakfast, lunch, dinner, bedtime, and in the middle of the night (if you are awake). In addition to liberal amounts of neutral foods (lean protein, healthy fat, neutral veggies), you have the option to eat a maximum of 5 grams of net carbs—what I call a "counter"—at breakfast, lunch, dinner, bedtime, or the middle of the night.

NET CARBS

To determine how many net carbs are in your food, check the nutrition facts label for total carbs and dietary fiber, then use this simple formula:

Total carb grams − dietary fiber grams = net carb grams

(For more on determining net carb grams, see page 146).

You must check nutrition facts for net carb grams for these low-carb foods, and all counters must have no more than 5 grams net carb/serving:

- Low-carb bread
- Low-carb wraps
- 1 cup popcorn
- Crackers in the quantity that nets 5 grams
- Low-carb milk
- Low-carb yogurt
- Greek or plain yogurt
- Low-carb protein shakes
- Low-carb juice
- Dark chocolate with more than 60 percent cacao (5 grams net carb)
- low-carb tortillas
- low-carb bread crumbs

If you cannot find these foods in your local grocery store, try looking for online purveyors that will deliver to your home. These online sites will provide the nutrition facts for their products, and you can choose the items that fit into your net carb parameters by following the easy formula above.

---

*All of these items must be run through the net carb formula and must fit into the 5 gram counter rule.

- Keep your counters about four to five hours apart.
- You can skip these treats, but you cannot save them up for later.
- Counters cannot be used as snacks between your meals.
- Snacks (except for bedtime and middle of the night) must be neutral foods only.

In Step 1, it is important to limit net carbs to a maximum of one counter at a meal. If you consume more than 5 grams of net carbs at a meal, bedtime, or middle of the night, the carb grams will add up, and your blood sugar will spike.

THE NUMBERS
TELL THE STORY

Identifying net carb grams is important on the Diabetes Miracle program. But you need to watch the nutrition labels in order to do so. Some companies have been known to use marketing tricks by putting misleading information on their packaging in an attempt to persuade you to buy their product. Recently, I've seen packages with such meaningless terms as "net effective carbs." Be careful: such phrases as *low carb*, *sugar-free*, *reduced sugar*, *carb-controlled*, and *diabetes-friendly* do not necessarily mean it's right for the Diabetes Miracle. Never rely on the marketing slogans, and don't be confused by all the numbers and percentages on the nutrition facts label.

The Diabetes Miracle lifestyle focuses on only three numbers on the label: serving size, total carbohydrate grams, and dietary fiber grams. (Naturally, anyone with food allergies or intolerances will also want to check the product's ingredient list.)

Nutrition Facts

Serving Size 2 tortillas (51g)
Servings Per Container 6

Amount Per Serving

Calories 110   Calories from Fat 10

% Daily Value*

Total Fat 1g	2%
Saturated Fat 0g	0%
Trans Fat 0g	
Cholesterol 0mg	0%
Sodium 30mg	1%
Total Carbohydrate 22g	7%
Dietary Fiber 2g	9%
Sugars 0g	
Protein 2g	

Vitamin A 0%	•	Vitamin C 0%
Calcium 2%	•	Iron 4%

*Percent Daily Values are based on a 2,000 calorie diet. Your daily values may be higher or lower depending on your calorie needs:

	Calories:	2,000	2,500
Total Fat	Less than	65g	80g
Saturated Fat	Less than	20g	25g
Cholesterol	Less than	300mg	300mg
Sodium	Less than	2,400mg	2,400mg
Total Carbohydrate		300g	375g
Dietary Fiber		25g	30g

Calories per gram:
Fat 9 • Carbohydrate 4 • Protein 4

*Reprinted from Nutridata.com.

It will take you less than thirty seconds to determine if the counter you are considering fits the Miracle parameter of 5 grams of carb or less:

Check serving size. Be careful because serving sizes can be deceptive. For example, many bottle beverages have serving sizes of 8 ounces when the bottle contains 24 ounces. This means you would get three times the carbs listed if you chose to drink the entire bottle. Companies sometimes do this to make their product appear healthier than it truly is.

Next, find total carbohydrate grams. The phrase **total carbohydrate** is always in bold type. Underneath this term, slightly indented, will be such entries as dietary fiber, sugar, sugar alcohol, and "other carb" grams. The total carbohydrate is the sum total of every carbohydrate gram in a serving of that particular food.*

Last, subtract dietary fiber grams. If the food choice contains dietary fiber, it will be listed right underneath total carbohydrate. You will need to subtract the dietary fiber grams from the total carbohydrate grams to find the net carbohydrate grams. Dietary fiber is the only part of the total carbohydrate grams that will not convert into blood sugar and affect insulin. The fiber will pass right through your body without converting to blood sugar. So, you get to subtract it away.

---

*Don't be fooled by looking at percentages to the right of grams on the label. Look at the total carb grams only.

LOW-CARB BREAD

Serving size: 1 slice
Total carbohydrate: 12 grams
Dietary fiber: 8 grams
Sugar alcohol: 1 gram
Other carbs: 3 grams

Total Carbohydrate: 12 grams
Minus dietary fiber: 8 grams
Net carbs: 4 grams

This bread fits into the counter zone at only 4 grams of net carbs.

Remember that in Step 1, if you are opting to add a 5 gram counter at breakfast, lunch, dinner, bedtime, or middle of the night, one slice of this bread would work at any of the allotted times, but two slices at once (a total of 8 grams net carbs) would be excessive and would cause insulin release.*

PORTION SIZES OF NEUTRAL FOODS . . . HOW MUCH IS RIGHT?

Because calories are not the focus of the Diabetes Miracle program, you don't have to be overly anxious about exactly how much of the neutral foods you are eating. Nonetheless, portion control will help you to remain on track. Following are some examples of sensible versus excessive versus inadequate portions:

- Sensible: a handful of peanuts three or four times throughout the day
- Excessive: 1 pound of peanuts per day

---

*For those following the Diabetes Miracle in countries other than the United States, please check with your nutrition labeling. Many European countries subtract fiber from their total carbohydrate grams and then show the dietary fiber again separately.

- Inadequate: fifteen peanuts per day

- Sensible: about 3 Tbsp of light ranch dressing on your garden salad
- Excessive: ¾ cup light ranch dressing on your garden salad
- Inadequate: 1 level tsp of light ranch dressing on your garden salad

- Sensible: ¾ cup low-fat cottage cheese mid-afternoon
- Excessive: 2 cups of low-fat cottage cheese mid-afternoon
- Inadequate: ¼ cup low-fat cottage cheese mid-afternoon

- Sensible: a 6-ounce sirloin burger at dinner
- Excessive: Four 6-ounce sirloin burgers at dinner
- Inadequate: a 2-ounce sirloin burger at dinner.

People who count out fifteen peanuts, level one teaspoon of salad dressing, or fret about the size of their sirloin burger err on the side of starvation. On the Diabetes Miracle program, fat loss is accomplished through hormonal balance. In order to achieve a pancreas/liver rest, there is a necessary period of restricting high-impact carb foods. We are left with protein, healthy fat, neutral vegetables, and an option of a 5 gram counter carb on Step 1. If you eliminate the most powerful carbohydrate, and then undereat your neutral options, you may deprive your body of adequate energy. Taking in too few calories will slow your metabolism and actually impede weight loss. Your body begins to hoard what you consume in an effort to keep you alive longer. In order to lose the right amount of fat on the Diabetes Miracle, you have to realize that less is not more when it comes to neutrals on Step 1. On the other hand, grossly overeating neutral foods, such as snacking on an entire jar of natural peanut butter, will only add excess fat and protein to your system. Your body will burn the peanut butter's fat content before it can move on to burning your fat stores.

It's all about moderation. Being overly conservative or overly liberal with neutral foods will work against you in terms of weight loss. Don't overthink it.

The solution is pretty simple. When you are hungry on Step 1, it is OK to eat. Eat foods from the neutral arrows at any time. When you feel full, stop eating. There is no reason to eat more than you normally would just because the food is neutral. Simply eat normally, keep your carbs in check, and you will soon see and feel the wonderful benefits of this program.

Taking It to the Extreme

Theresa just turned 62 years of age and was tired of how she looked and felt. She had always been a looker and couldn't believe the image she now saw in her mirror.

The woman who looked back at her appeared older than 62, tired, bloated, and pale. Her hair was thin and lacked luster. Her skin was a bit ashen. Her weight had gravitated to around her middle, and she had a roll that stood out further than her chest. She was told that her blood sugar was slightly elevated (although she was never told the reading), and she was taking medication for blood pressure along with an antidepressant.

She quickly read only the diet and exercise piece of the Diabetes Miracle program, went shopping, and began the program the next morning.

Every morning she stepped on her scale. Let's be honest, three or four times a day, every day, she stepped on her scale. One day the weight was up, the next it was down, then up, then it stayed the same, then down, down, up. Theresa was flummoxed. It didn't make any sense.

She thought, "Maybe I'm missing something." The next morning she got out of bed and stepped onto the elliptical machine. Theresa had not exercised in years. She stayed on for an hour. Her muscles ached and burned. She felt awful. From that day on, she decided she just couldn't exercise. She stopped all exercising and cut down on her portions of neutral foods. I must be overeating, she reasoned. She counted out ten almonds, measured 1 level tablespoon of natural peanut butter, and weighed 3 ounce portions of chicken. She decided not to use 5 gram counters as they were just extra calories.

Day after day, the scale lagged. Theresa ate less and less, but the scale didn't budge. She was frustrated and annoyed and fumed, "This program doesn't work. Nothing is happening."

A few weeks later, Theresa bumped into her friend Alexa. She looked amazing. She had lost what looked like twenty pounds, she was wearing stylish clothes, and she was glowing. "I'm following the Miracle program," she explained. She went on to say that she takes a one-hour walk first thing in the morning five times a week but always has one-half a banana before she begins and the other half at the thirty-minute mark.

She raved about how she loved the freedom to eat neutral foods liberally. She never counted nuts, measured nut butter, or paid close attention to her portions of lean protein. She ate until she was full and never felt hungry.

She was careful to drink 64 ounces of liquid a day to rid her body of the breakdown products of fat. She lost within her expected target range and realized that her eleven pounds of fat loss looked like a twenty-pound loss.

She had tons of energy and felt so much younger than her 55 years. She recommended that Theresa try the program.

Theresa went home, put her scale in the garage, and began to follow the program to the letter—ultimately to the results she wanted.

ADJUSTING AFTER A SLIP-UP

If you slip up on Step 1, you will have to make adjustments. For every five-hour block that contains errors while you are on Step 1, you must add on three days after the end of the eight-week period. For example: If you are celebrating a birthday and for dinner you have a tossed salad with dressing, lasagna, a slice of garlic bread, and a taste of birthday cake, and the meal is happening during one five-hour period, you will need to add on three full days after the end of the eighth week.

If, on your birthday, you had a bagel for breakfast; a slice of pizza for lunch; and turkey with dressing, whipped potatoes, green beans, and birthday cake for dinner, then you had slip-ups in three separate five-hour blocks. This would set your program back nine days.

Step 1 is meant to be a time of rest and rehab. When you go off program, it really engages the pancreas. Your blood sugar will quickly rise, the pancreas will snap to attention and over-release insulin, and your liver will begin to refill with glycogen. It will take three days to right every five-hour-block slip-up.

Another problem with slip-ups in Step 1 is that cravings, fatigue, irritability, nausea, light-headedness, and other symptoms will occur because you are shocking your system. Be extra vigilant with diet restrictions during that three-day cleanup because you will be tempted to slip up again.

ARE NATURAL SUGARS HEALTHIER THAN ARTIFICIAL SWEETENERS?

Many people mistakenly believe that because a sweetener is natural, it must be healthy. Using sugar, agave nectar, honey, or other sugars for sweetening is not recommended on the Diabetes Miracle. These sweeteners have a high glycemic index, meaning they will spike blood sugar almost instantaneously. Instead, try a sugar substitute, such as sucralose or stevia.

Remember that a person with prediabetes or type 2 diabetes has a physiological condition that, when unchecked, results in wide swings in blood sugar, fat deposits in and on the body, chronic health conditions, and sapped energy. Sugar, honey, and agave are all simple carbohydrates that exacerbate that condition by causing an immediate, sharp rise in blood sugar, which triggers the pancreas and causes insulin imbalance.

Consider that one tablespoon of honey contains 15 grams of high-glycemic carb (15 grams in one level tablespoon). Did you know that 1 level tablespoon of sugar has the same amount? Remember that all carbs break down to blood sugar, and a packet of sugar and honey are very quick-acting carbs.

HIGH-FRUCTOSE CORN SYRUP? POISON OR HYPE?

High-fructose corn syrup (HFCS) has been maligned as a toxic substance used to sweeten beverages, sodas, baked goods, and processed foods. It is also known simply as corn syrup.

In the same way that sugar and honey quickly turn to blood sugar and wreak havoc on the metabolism of those with diabetes, so does any excess fruit sugar, corn sugar, beet sugar, and so on. High-fructose corn syrup has been singled out and blamed for such health problems as childhood obesity, high triglycerides, dental cavities, poor nutrition, and heart disease. If we were instead adding maple syrup or beet syrup to beverages, baked goods, and processed foods, children with Met B would experience excess insulin release, fat production, dental caries, and heart disease. There is insufficient evidence to say that corn syrup is less healthy than are other types of added sweeteners.

It doesn't matter whether the sweetening ingredient is derived from sugarcane, beet sugar, corn sugar, or fruit sugar—as the commercial says, sugar is sugar. If you are avoiding HFCS and using agave nectar or honey, you are still consuming high-glycemic carbs.

How to Sweeten on Step 1

If you desire, you can use 1 level teaspoon of sugar (a packet) or 1 teaspoon of honey as your 5 gram counter at any meal, but this packet of sugar would take the place of a nutritious, healthful food, such as a 5 gram carb wrap (tortilla), a piece of low-carb bread, ½ cup Greek yogurt, or a low-carb protein shake. These foods also give you a feeling of satiety—many contain appreciable fiber too.

Of the sugar replacements currently available, I am personally inclined to choose stevia or sucralose. You needn't count the carb grams in either because they are not absorbed like carbohydrate and don't influence blood sugar and insulin response. (Although aspartame and saccharin are approved by the Food and Drug Administration and can fit into the guidelines of the Diabetes Miracle, they are not my personal choices.)

Just as I don't recommend excessive intake of neutral foods, I don't recommend excessive use of nonnutritive sweeteners. I generally limit my own use of sugar replacements to about two servings per day on average; I might sweeten my morning coffee with sucralose and have a sugar-free beverage later in the day.

ALCOHOL

If you have been diagnosed with prediabetes or type 2 diabetes, it would be prudent to get your physician's recommendation on the use of alcohol. Everyone's medical profile is different, and there may be conditions, medications, or circumstances other than your blood sugar that may contradict alcohol consumption.

Because wine is derived from grapes and most liquors and light beer are made from grains, people tend to believe that they will cause an immediate rise in blood sugar. After all, grapes and regular bread are not allowed on Step 1 of the program. Although it is true that wine, light beer, and most liquors begin as carbs, the fermentation and distillation process changes the chemical structure of these ingredients so that they metabolize through the fat pathway rather than the carbohydrate pathway.

With the exception of sweetened mixed drinks, sweetened liquors, dessert wines, liqueurs, port wine, and sangria, you will not count most wines or liquors—such as gin, whiskey, vodka, wine, champagne, and light beer—as carbohydrates on the Diabetes Miracle.

That said, there are some things you'll want to keep in mind should you decide to drink alcohol while on Step 1. The liver is the detox factory of the body. During Step 1, your liver is resting and working at a relaxed pace. As a result, the alcohol content from your first drink may remain at a higher than normal concentration in your system when you have your next drink. The alcohol essentially stacks up in your system. As a result, you can expect to feel tipsy sooner than usual when drinking alcohol on Step 1 and you should pace your drinking.

The maximum recommended amount of alcohol (with physician approval only) is one to two drinks. One drink is defined as 5 ounces of wine, 1 ½ ounces of liquor, or 12 ounces of light beer.

Be aware that many wine glasses are more like water goblets, and your local bar's shot of liquor may contain 3 ounces. In some circumstances, you may think you've had two glasses of wine when in fact you've had three. Remember to check the carbohydrate content of the mixers you add to alcohol-containing drinks. Choose sugar-free tonic water, sugar-free soda, low-carb juice (with 1 gram net carb or less in 4 ounces), seltzer water, or sugar-free drink mixes (make sure to read the label for carb content of sugar-free items).

ALCOHOL'S IMPACT ON MORNING FASTING BLOOD READINGS

Although alcohol starts out as carbohydrate, it is processed in your body similarly to fat and does not cause an immediate rise in blood sugar. People are often surprised when they check their two-hour post-meal reading after drinking wine with the meal: The wine didn't make a big difference in their blood sugar.

Oddly, if you have type 2 diabetes, you may find that your fasting reading is elevated the morning after an evening that included alcohol. Although your two-hour post-meal reading after dinner with several glasses of wine may have been normal, you may experience an unusually high morning reading.

The liver has many functions in the body, and when several jobs need to happen at once, it prioritizes their importance. The liver is not only the detox organ; when you go beyond five hours without eating, the liver also will step up to the plate and self-feed. When a person drinks a larger quantity of alcohol, the liver sets detox as its main priority and goes about the business of cleaning the blood of this toxin. As a result, the self-feeding mechanism takes a back seat.

If a person takes medication to lower blood sugar (oral medication or insulin), the medication continues to work during the night. On a night not including alcohol, the liver would self-feed, and there would be blood sugar status quo. But if the liver is working overtime to clean up alcohol, self-feeding takes a back seat to alcohol detox. It is possible to have low blood sugar in the middle of the night, and when the liver finishes cleaning the alcohol, it may overreact to push the blood sugar up. As a result, morning blood sugar readings can be out of control.

Limit alcoholic drinks, with physician's permission and based on your own medical conditions and medications, to a maximum of one or two in a day, taken with food. Make sure to take an appropriate snack prior to going to bed. Also, monitor blood sugar to see what effect your alcohol consumption has on your blood sugar because every body is different.

SAMPLE MENUS FOR STEP 1

BREAKFAST

Omelet with shredded low-fat cheddar, diced bell peppers, and
  onions
One slice low-carb toast (5 gram counter)
Whipped butter and zero-carb strawberry jelly
Coffee with half-and-half and sucralose

Low-fat cottage cheese
Tomato wedges and bell pepper slices
Five multigrain wheat crackers (5 gram counter)
Tea with stevia

4 ounces tomato juice or vegetable juice
Low-carb wrap (5 gram counter) filled with thinly sliced ham and
  low-fat cheddar (microwave to melt cheese, if desired)
Green tea with stevia or sucralose

Low-carb chocolate, vanilla, or strawberry protein shake (5 gram
  counter)
Handful of natural almonds
Water with lemon

Dip of part-skim ricotta cheese mixed with ¼ tsp of vanilla, ½ tsp
  sucralose or stevia, ½ tsp cinnamon
Sprinkle with a handful of chopped pecans
Herbal tea with lemon

Scrambled eggs or egg whites
Two strips of turkey bacon
One slice low-carb toast (5 gram counter)
Whipped butter
Coffee with creamer and sucralose

Low-carb yogurt or ½ cup Greek yogurt (5 gram counter)
Celery sticks with natural peanut or almond butter
Water with lime and stevia

Store-bought or homemade quiche (remove all crust or
     prepare/purchase crustless)
One slice low-carb toast (5 gram counter)
Whipped butter
Unsweetened almond milk

Poached egg on top of one slice low-carb toast (5 gram counter)
Coffee with half and half (cream) and stevia

Scoop of low-fat cottage or ricotta cheese
Whole-grain crackers in a 5 gram amount (5 gram counter)
Carb-free jelly
Natural almond butter
Decaf coffee with light creamer

Low-carb wrap (5 gram counter) spread with whipped cream
     cheese or natural almond butter and carb-free jelly. Roll tightly.
     Cut the roll into eight bit-size slices
Green tea with lemon

LUNCH

Low-carb wrap (5 gram counter) filled with tuna, egg, shrimp,
     chicken, or ham salad (light mayo or small amount of regular
     mayo)
Lettuce and tomato slices
Cheesy chips (place "chip-size" piles [about 1 Tbsp/pile] of grated
     cheddar cheese on a baking pan in a 400 degree preheated oven

(continued)

until they get golden brown. Check them frequently. Cool and remove from baking tray).
Herbal iced tea with stevia and lemon

Turkey salad on a bed of lettuce and tomato wedges
Sugar-free gelatin cup with a swirl of light whipped cream
Water with lemon wedge

Leftover grilled chicken, cubed low-fat cheddar cheese
Sliced avocado
Romaine lettuce and tomato slices in a low-carb wrap
    (5 gram counter); spread with light sour cream
Diet soda

Hot and sour soup or egg drop soup
Steamed chicken, shrimp, beef, or pork
Steamed vegetables (broccoli, scallions, onions, water chestnuts)
Chicken broth or some of your egg drop soup (use as a sauce over
    the chicken/veggies)
Soy sauce (if desired)
Green tea

Grilled cheeseburger patty wrapped in a lettuce leaf and served
    with tomato, onion, and low-carb ketchup
1 cup popcorn (5 gram counter)
Sparkling water with lemon

Cobb salad (grilled chicken strips, crisp turkey bacon, shredded
    cheddar cheese, sliced eggs, and avocado layered over a base of
    chopped romaine lettuce)
Light ranch dressing

(continued)

Baked tortilla chips (that equal 5 grams net carbs)

Water with lime wedge

Restaurant chicken, beef, or shrimp fajitas (just skip the tortilla
   shells!)

Low-carb wrap (5 gram counter)

Diet soda with lemon wedge

Tuna salad on a bed of romaine

Whole-grain crackers in an amount that equals a 5 gram counter

Flavored seltzer water

DINNER

5 ounces white wine

Grilled chicken breast topped with marinara sauce (tomatoes and
   herbs/spices only) and melted mozzarella cheese

Mashed cauliflower (steam or boil cauliflower until soft and mash
   or whip with butter, adding salt/pepper to taste)

Garden salad with balsamic vinaigrette

Decaf coffee with creamer

Square of 60 percent dark chocolate in a 5 gram net carb amount
   (5 gram counter)

Grilled sirloin steak

Sautéed onions and mushrooms

Broccoli spears with grated parmesan

Sugar-free gelatin with light whipped topping

Sparkling water

85 percent lean burger with cheese, served open faced on low-carb
    bread (5 gram counter)
Lettuce, tomato slices, and onion
Low-carb ketchup
Side Caesar salad without croutons
Flavored seltzer water

Omelet with ham, cheese, and veggies
One slice low-carb toast (5 gram counter)
Natural almond butter
Decaf tea with lemon

Glass of red wine
Shirataki noodles (soy noodles from the organic refrigerator
    section)
½ cup marinara sauce (no sugar added)
Parmesan cheese
One slice of low-carb bread toasted and spread with garlic butter (5
    gram counter)
Italian garden salad
Water with lemon

Broiled or grilled shrimp
Spinach salad with vinaigrette, olives, and feta cheese
Baked tortilla chips that equal 5 grams net carbs (5 gram counter)
½ cup salsa
Lemon water

Roast turkey breast
Gravy (check label for 5 gram carb amount)
Whipped or mashed cauliflower (use instead of mashed potatoes)
Green beans Florentine

Ricotta dessert: mix ricotta cheese with carb-free chocolate syrup
and top with whipped cream and chopped walnuts
Iced tea with lemon and stevia

Dip of cottage cheese mixed with ¼ cup blueberries (5 gram carb
counter)
One handful of cocoa-roasted almonds (check ingredients for no
added sugar)
Decaf coffee with creamer

Fill a low-carb wrap (5 gram counter) with grilled chicken strips or
sautéed cubed tofu, shredded cheddar, sautéed peppers, and
onions. Add shredded lettuce, diced fresh tomato, and avocado.
Drizzle with light ranch dressing
Cheesy chips
Lemon water

Chopped garden salad with balsamic vinaigrette
Broiled flounder
Broccoli spears with lemon pepper
5 gram frozen pop (5 gram counter).

STEP 1 SNACKS

These neutral snacks can be used on any step of the Diabetes
Miracle:
Low-fat cheese
Olives
Celery with natural peanut butter
Nuts
Low-carb protein shakes with less than 2 grams net carbs
Boiled egg

Ricotta dessert (ricotta cheese mixed with sucralose or stevia, and
  either vanilla extract, almond extract, lemon extract, or carb-free
  chocolate syrup to taste. Serve chilled)
Sugar-free gelatin with whipped topping
Spoonful of peanut or almond butter
Ham or turkey and cheese roll-ups
Allowed neutral veggies with low-fat dip (sour cream and
  herbs/seasonings)
Edamame
Sunflower or pumpkin seeds
Soy nuts
Cheesy chips

FREQUENTLY ASKED QUESTIONS FOR STEP 1

*I have type 2 diabetes, and my most recent hemoglobin A1C was
6.2. I take an oral medication that lowers my blood sugar. I realize
that given my good A1C, I should expect to feel tired, hungry, irritable, and experience cravings during the first three to four days of
Step 1. Well, it's Day 7, and I'm following the program by the
book, but I am finding myself feeling dizzy, sweaty, extremely hungry, and weak.*

You say that you are following the dietary guidelines of Step 1. You
began the program with reasonable A1C and you started Step 1 taking
oral medication to lower blood sugar. Have you checked your blood
sugar when you are experiencing these symptoms? By Day 7 of the
program, it is very possible that you are already experiencing lower
blood sugar on your current dose of medication. The next time you
feel these symptoms, check your blood sugar. If it is under 70, you are
hypoglycemic. Treat the hypoglycemia (see pages 294–295) and inform your doctor, who can make a decision about your medication.

*I have type 2 diabetes and began the Diabetes Miracle with a he-
moglobin A1C of 10.6. I take oral medications during the day, and
my physician recently added a single dose of long-acting insulin at
night. It's Day 7, I'm following the program by the book, but I am
finding myself dizzy, sweaty, extremely hungry, and weak. I thought
I was having hypoglycemia, so I checked my blood sugar and was
surprised to see that it was normal at 120, 117, 124. I realize that
I'm not hypoglycemic, but I sure feel it.*

You certainly did begin the program with very elevated blood sugar;
for the past three months your average blood glucose was 300 mg/dL.
As a result of a long period of high readings, your body got accustomed
to functioning at this unhealthy level. Now that your readings are significantly better, your brain is misreading normal blood sugar as low.

It is wonderful that you tested your blood sugar when you felt hypoglycemic. It is also great that you noted that the readings were not reg-
istering hypoglycemia. If you treated the feeling of hypoglycemia, you
would have boosted your sugar back into the 300 range. Your body
would say "ahhhh, that's better," because unfortunately, 300 blood
sugar is what your body has become accustomed to.

In short order, your new bar will be set, and you will feel normal at
such readings as 120. Until then, test before assuming it's hypoglycemia.

*Do I have to have a 5 gram carb counter at each meal, at bedtime,
and in the middle of the night?*

No. The 5 gram counters are optional. Some people ignore these
carbs completely, but I am not one of those people. Whether you
choose to include the 5 gram counters or not, your progress will be the
same in Step 1.

Remember, if you choose not to use a counter at one meal, you can't save it for the next and add it to that meal's counter. This would stack the carb grams, raise blood sugar, trigger insulin release, and slow weight loss.

You have the option to use a 5 gram counter at breakfast, lunch, dinner, bedtime and in the middle of the night if you are awake.

> *I am in Week 5 of Step 1. I have type 2 diabetes, and I take no medication. Since Day 5 of the program, my readings had been normal. I looked great and felt great. Then, my girlfriends and I went away for a "Ladies-Only Weekend." I was doing fine on Step 1 until the last evening, when I had some bread, a little pasta, and a few spoons of dessert. Do I have to go back and start all over again?*

Take a deep breath. You put five weeks into Step 1. You had a break in one five-hour period. All you need do is add three days to the end of your eight weeks. Be careful, though. When you break the peace and tranquility of Step 1, you are more inclined to cave again as cravings return. Get your resolve back and move forward.

> *I found these great cookies marked "low-carb" and "sugar-free." Can I have them on Step 1? I looked at the sugar grams, and they show 0 grams of sugar.*

The only way to make a decision about a product on Step 1 is to look at the nutrition facts label on the package (see page 145). Note the serving size, and then calculate the net carbs: Total carb grams-dietary fiber grams = net carbs. If you come up with 5 grams or less net carbs, you can use the proper number of cookies as a counter at a meal, at bedtime, or in the middle of the night if you are awake. Don't let the food company do the math for you. Some companies will make up their own formulas and use their own terminology to make the product appear healthy.

Also, the sugar grams on a food label refer only to the grams of table sugar in the product. Food companies are crafty in sweetening their products with sugar alcohols, fructose, HFCS, and other types of sugar, so they needn't list these grams next to the word sugar. Remember, the Miracle program does not require that you look at sugar grams—just total carb grams minus dietary fiber.*

What can I do about constipation on Step 1?

1. As you know, having prediabetes or diabetes increases your chances of becoming dehydrated. Drink a minimum of 64 ounces of decaf fluid or water every day to prevent constipation. It doesn't matter when you drink the water as long as you've taken in 64 ounces by the day's end.

   Although caffeine is allowed on the Diabetes Miracle plan, don't count caffeine-containing beverages toward your fluid requirement. However, decaf fluids do count.

2. You can also increase your fiber intake. Make sure to use a lot of raw veggies, salads, nuts, and low-carb breads and wraps as your 5 gram counters. Some people choose to add 1 heaping teaspoon of powdered plant fiber that dissolves in liquid to each meal. This adds about 5 grams of fiber. By increasing fiber intake and drinking adequate fluid, your stool will be bulkier, and your bowel movements will be more regular.

---

* Total Carb Grams: 7g
  Dietary fiber: 3g
  Sugar alcohol: 2g
  Other carbs: 2g

3. Some people find that when they add two green tea bags/day, their problems with constipation are over. Make sure you are drinking your green tea daily.

4. Physical activity, especially walking, helps to move that gastrointestinal tract in the right direction—as does gravity. Stand up and move around, and you will coax that colon into moving.

5. You can also try this old standby: First thing in the morning and last thing at night, add the juice of 1 lemon to a cup of herbal tea. Drink warm.

I notice that the natural peanut butter, cottage cheese, and almonds I buy contain carb grams. Do I have to count these carb grams toward my 5 gram counter?

Foods listed in the protein, fat, and neutral vegetable arrows on pages 138–139 do not normally need to have label checks or be measured for portion control. As for portion size, be reasonably liberal with these foods. Because of the mechanics of Step 1, you must purposely eliminate impact carbohydrate foods. If you severely limit your healthy protein and fat intake (neutral foods), you can slow your metabolism and slow weight loss. That said, let common sense prevail. The Diabetes Miracle is a blood sugar–stabilizing, fat-burning lifestyle program. Don't overconsume neutral foods just because they are neutral. Eat them when you are hungry, but don't overdo. If your intake is excessive in fat, you will waste time burning the fat from food rather than the fat from you.

I couldn't resist and weighed myself after only two weeks on the program. Although I feel better and my blood sugar is now excellent, the scale hasn't moved.

Losing weight with Met B, prediabetes, or type 2 diabetes is much different from normal weight loss. On a calorie-based diet, a person loses pounds that are composed of water weight, muscle loss, and fat loss. Calorie-based programs are based on an actual formula: calories in – calories out = weight. A person losing weight by counting calories will lose weight in a methodical style: lose a few pounds, plateau, lose a few pounds, plateau.

A person with Met B doesn't have a calorie issue; she has a hormonal imbalance. On this plan, you are not counting and burning calories; you are balancing blood sugar and insulin release. Each person will respond differently because of her own physiology. Your weight loss is never methodical, but at the end of the eight weeks, it will be within target range.

I advise you to weigh and measure yourself at the beginning of every eight-week period.* Don't bother with weigh-ins or remeasures during the days or weeks between. When you follow the dietary guidelines, exercise as directed, drink adequate fluid, take the recommended vitamins and minerals, and eat throughout the day, you will lose exactly the right amount of fat. But you will look as though you have lost twice as much weight. Be patient; this program works. In addition to the expected pounds of fat, your pounds lost and inches lost every eight weeks will be very close. If you lose 15 pounds in eight weeks of Step 1, and it is all fat loss, you will lose just about 15 inches. On a calorie-based diet, a 15-pound weight loss causes only a 7- to 8-inch loss. On the Miracle program, you are losing all fat, and fat loss has major volume.

How can I be sure that the pounds I am losing are all fat? I lost within the expected amount, but how do I know that it's not fat, muscle, and water?

---

*The measurement chart (page 335) shows you the areas to measure and then remeasure after eight weeks. Add up the inches lost, and you will have a snapshot of your total inches lost to compare against pounds lost.

On a calorie-based weight-loss program, a 10-pound loss usually results in a 5-inch loss. On the Diabetes Miracle, a 10-pound loss usually enables a 9- to11-inch loss. The Diabetes Miracle is not a calorie-counting program; it is working on regulating the hormone insulin. If you incorporate thirty minutes of physical activity over and above your normal daily activity for five days a week and drink adequate water, the program targets fat loss.

With the Diabetes Miracle, it's not just pounds lost. It's important that the pounds lost and the inches lost are simpatico. To determine if the pounds you are losing are mainly fat pounds, after every eight-week period, note the pounds lost. From the pounds lost number, the range of inch loss you can expect will be from minus 1 to plus 1 of the number of pounds lost.

If you lost 10 pounds and only 7-inches, you can assume that you lost about 7 pounds of fat tissue and 2–3 pounds of muscle or water.

After eight weeks, compare your fat loss to the guidelines below. At the end of each eight-week period in Steps 1 and 2, you should have met the anticipated fat-loss target. If done correctly, you will not lose muscle or water; you will lose only fat, both in the form of cholesterol and of body fat.

The following tables will show you how many fat pounds you can expect to lose after eight weeks on Steps 1 or 2.

What if I don't lose weight within your target range?

Unlike typical calorie-based weight-loss diets, the pounds lost on the Diabetes Miracle program should come entirely from fat loss. It is not recommended that you lose more weight or less than the chart indicates. A body of a 45-year-old male who is 5 feet 11 inches and weighs 245 pounds can only lose a certain amount of fat in eight weeks. Losing more weight than the chart indicates is not good. It means you lost fat plus muscle and water. If you lose less than the expected amount,

FAT-LOSS EXPECTATIONS DURING STEPS ONE AND TWO

WOMEN

Find your height and starting weight in the left-hand columns to identify the number of "fat" pounds that you are expected to lose during the upcoming eight weeks during Step 1 or 2. Remember, you will look like you have lost twice as much weight.

4'10"	90–130 lbs.	= 3–5 lbs. fat loss	5'6"	130–170 lbs.	= 3–5 lbs. fat loss
	130–170 lbs.	= 6–13 lbs. fat loss		170–210 lbs.	= 6–13 lbs. fat loss
	170–210 lbs.	= 14–21 lbs. fat loss		210–250 lbs.	= 14–21 lbs. fat loss
	210–250 lbs.	= 22–29 lbs. fat loss		250–290 lbs.	= 22–29 lbs. fat loss
4'11"	95–135 lbs.	= 3–5 lbs. fat loss	5'7"	135–175 lbs.	= 3–5 lbs. fat loss
	135–175 lbs.	= 6–13 lbs. fat loss		175–215 lbs.	= 6–13 lbs. fat loss
	175–215 lbs.	= 14–21 lbs. fat loss		215–255 lbs.	= 14–21 lbs. fat loss
	215–255 lbs.	= 22–29 lbs. fat loss		255–295 lbs.	= 22–29 lbs. fat loss
5'0"	100–140 lbs.	= 3–5 lbs. fat loss	5'8"	140–180 lbs.	= 3–5 lbs. fat loss
	140–180 lbs.	= 6–13 lbs. fat loss		180–220 lbs.	= 6–13 lbs. fat loss
	180–220 lbs.	= 14–21 lbs. fat loss		220–260 lbs.	= 14–21 lbs. fat loss
	220–260 lbs.	= 22–29 lbs. fat loss		260–300 lbs.	= 22–29 lbs. fat loss
5'1"	105–145 lbs.	= 3–5 lbs. fat loss	5'9"	145–185 lbs.	= 3–5 lbs. fat loss
	145–185 lbs.	= 6–13 lbs. fat loss		185–225 lbs.	= 6–13 lbs. fat loss
	185–225 lbs.	= 14–21 lbs. fat loss		225–265 lbs.	= 14–21 lbs. fat loss
	225–265 lbs.	= 22–29 lbs. fat loss		265–305 lbs.	= 22–29 lbs. fat loss
5'2"	110–150 lbs.	= 3–5 lbs. fat loss	5'10"	150–190 lbs.	= 3–5 lbs. fat loss
	150–190 lbs.	= 6–13 lbs. fat loss		190–230 lbs.	= 6–13 lbs. fat loss
	190–230 lbs.	= 14–21 lbs. fat loss		230–270 lbs.	= 14–21 lbs. fat loss
	230–270 lbs.	= 22–29 lbs. fat loss		270–310 lbs.	= 22–29 lbs. fat loss
5'3"	115–155 lbs.	= 3–5 lbs. fat loss	5'11"	155–195 lbs.	= 3–5 lbs. fat loss
	155–195 lbs.	= 6–13 lbs. fat loss		195–235 lbs.	= 6–13 lbs. fat loss
	195–235 lbs.	= 14–21 lbs. fat loss		235–275 lbs.	= 14–21 lbs. fat loss
	235–275 lbs.	= 22–29 lbs. fat loss		275–315 lbs.	= 22–29 lbs. fat loss
5'4"	120–160 lbs.	= 3–5 lbs. fat loss	6'0"	160–200 lbs.	= 3–5 lbs. fat loss
	160–200 lbs.	= 6–13 lbs. fat loss		200–240 lbs.	= 6–13 lbs. fat loss
	200–240 lbs.	= 14–21 lbs. fat loss		240–280 lbs.	= 14–21 lbs. fat loss
	240–280 lbs.	= 22–29 lbs. fat loss		280–320 lbs.	= 22–29 lbs. fat loss
5'5"	125–165 lbs.	= 3–5 lbs. fat loss			
	165–205 lbs.	= 6–13 lbs. fat loss			
	205–245 lbs.	= 14–21 lbs. fat loss			
	245–285 lbs.	= 22–29 lbs. fat loss			

MEN

Find your height and starting weight in the left-hand columns to identify the number of "fat" pounds that you are expected to lose during the upcoming eight weeks during Step 1 or 2. Remember, you will look like you have lost twice as much weight.

5'0"	106–146 lbs.	= 3–5 lbs. fat loss	5'8"	154–194 lbs.	= 3–5 lbs. fat loss
	146–186 lbs.	= 6–13 lbs. fat loss		194–234 lbs.	= 6–13 lbs. fat loss
	186–226 lbs.	= 14–21 lbs. fat loss		234–274 lbs.	= 14–21 lbs. fat loss
	226–266 lbs.	= 22–29 lbs. fat loss		274–314 lbs.	= 22–29 lbs. fat loss
5'1"	112–152 lbs.	= 3–5 lbs. fat loss	5'9"	160–200 lbs.	= 3–5 lbs. fat loss
	152–192 lbs.	= 6–13 lbs. fat loss		200–240 lbs.	= 6–13 lbs. fat loss
	192–232 lbs.	= 14–21 lbs. fat loss		240–280 lbs.	= 14–21 lbs. fat loss
	232–272 lbs.	= 22–29 lbs. fat loss		280–320 lbs.	= 22–29 lbs. fat loss
5'2"	118–158 lbs.	= 3–5 lbs. fat loss	5'10"	166–206 lbs.	= 3–5 lbs. fat loss
	158–198 lbs.	= 6–13 lbs. fat loss		206–246 lbs.	= 6–13 lbs. fat loss
	198–238 lbs.	= 14–21 lbs. fat loss		246–286 lbs.	= 14–21 lbs. fat loss
	238–278 lbs.	= 22–29 lbs. fat loss		286–326 lbs.	= 22–29 lbs. fat loss
5'3"	124–164 lbs.	= 3–5 lbs. fat loss	5'11"	172–212 lbs.	= 3–5 lbs. fat loss
	164–204 lbs.	= 6–13 lbs. fat loss		212–252 lbs.	= 6–13 lbs. fat loss
	204–244 lbs.	= 14–21 lbs. fat loss		252–292 lbs.	= 14–21 lbs. fat loss
	244–284 lbs.	= 22–29 lbs. fat loss		292–332 lbs.	= 22–29 lbs. fat loss
5'4"	130–170 lbs.	= 3–5 lbs. fat loss	6'0"	178–218 lbs.	= 3–5 lbs. fat loss
	170–210 lbs.	= 6–13 lbs. fat loss		218–258 lbs.	= 6–13 lbs. fat loss
	210–250 lbs.	= 14–21 lbs. fat loss		258–298 lbs.	= 14–21 lbs. fat loss
	250–290 lbs.	= 22–29 lbs. fat loss		298–338 lbs.	= 22–29 lbs. fat loss
5'5"	136–176 lbs.	= 3–5 lbs. fat loss	6'1"	184–224 lbs.	= 3–5 lbs. fat loss
	176–216 lbs.	= 6–13 lbs. fat loss		224–264 lbs.	= 6–13 lbs. fat loss
	216–256 lbs.	= 14–21 lbs. fat loss		264–304 lbs.	= 14–21 lbs. fat loss
	256–296 lbs.	= 22–29 lbs. fat loss		304–344 lbs.	= 22–29 lbs. fat loss
5'6"	142–182 lbs.	= 3–5 lbs. fat loss	6'2"	190–230 lbs.	= 3–5 lbs. fat loss
	182–222 lbs.	= 6–13 lbs. fat loss		230–270 lbs.	= 6–13 lbs. fat loss
	222–262 lbs.	= 14–21 lbs. fat loss		270–310 lbs.	= 14–21 lbs. fat loss
	262–302 lbs.	= 22–29 lbs. fat loss		310–350 lbs.	= 22–29 lbs. fat loss
5'7"	148–188 lbs.	= 3–5 lbs. fat loss	6'3"	196–236 lbs.	= 3–5 lbs. fat loss
	188–228 lbs.	= 6–13 lbs. fat loss		236–276 lbs.	= 6–13 lbs. fat loss
	228–268 lbs.	= 14–21 lbs. fat loss		276–316 lbs.	= 14–21 lbs. fat loss
	268–308 lbs.	= 22–29 lbs. fat loss		316–356 lbs.	= 22–29 lbs. fat loss

6'4"	202–242 lbs.	= 3–5 lbs. fat loss	6'6"	214–254 lbs.	= 3–5 lbs. fat loss
	242–282 lbs.	= 6–13 lbs. fat loss		254–294 lbs.	= 6–13 lbs. fat loss
	282–322 lbs.	= 14–21 lbs. fat loss		294–334 lbs.	= 14–21 lbs. fat loss
	322–362 lbs.	= 22=29 lbs. fat loss		334–374 lbs.	= 22–29 lbs. fat loss
6'5"	208–248 lbs.	= 3–5 lbs. fat loss			
	248–288 lbs.	= 6–13 lbs. fat loss			
	288–328 lbs.	= 14–21 lbs. fat loss			
	328–368 lbs.	= 22=29 lbs. fat loss			

it's not because you ate too much. If your fat loss is outside of the expected range, it's important to find the reason so you can solve it before moving on.

What if I lose more weight than the chart indicates?

It might seem fantastic to lose more than the charts indicate, but in the case of the Diabetes Miracle, this is not beneficial. If you lose more pounds than were expected, chances are you didn't lose mainly fat. You can verify this because your pounds lost will most likely exceed your inches lost after the eighth week. There are two primary reasons that a person will lose more weight than expected.

1. You followed the diet but did not exercise

A person who follows the Diabetes Miracle but does not exercise will actually lose more weight than a person who exercises as directed. I know this sounds like a mistake, but it is true. Again, remember that weight loss is much different from fat loss. Lack of exercise causes you to lose pounds of fat *and* pounds of valuable muscle. Losing muscle is not desirable because you lose valuable furnaces that actually serve to burn blood sugar and decrease your need for medication. Muscle also gives your body shape and tone.

Although it appears as if you did better by losing more weight, you did not lose more fat. Move that body! You must do a minimum of thirty minutes of physical activity over and above your normal day, four to five times per week to lower your blood sugar, preserve muscle, burn more fat, and retain strength and tone.

2. Inadequate water or decaffeinated fluid intake

If you fail to consume the recommended amount of water/decaf liquid, your extra weight loss may simply be a sign of dehydration. Drink a few glasses of water, and that scale will move up again. Water loss is a matter of drinking too little water. This is unhealthy for your kidneys and allows the sugar, minerals, waste products, and toxins in the blood to be in greater concentration.

What if I lose less weight than the chart indicates?

On a typical weight-loss diet based upon calories, a person who does not lose adequate weight is most likely overeating and underexercising. In the body of a person with Metabolism A, body weight is achieved by following a calories in/calories out formula—burn more calories than you take in, and you will lose weight. It's a different ball game with the Diabetes Miracle. On this lifestyle plan, it is possible to slow your fat loss by not eating enough neutral foods. There are seven primary reasons that a person will lose less weight than expected.

1. Are you overeating carbs or carb-stacking?

You may be consuming more carbohydrate than is recommended on the program. Remember, counter carbs are optional at meals, bedtime, or in the middle of the night. If you exceed this amount, your pancreas will respond with excess insulin, and weight loss will slow or stop. Also, if you are taking counter carbs between meals, your carb grams will stack and cause the pancreas to engage.

5 gram counter carbs . . . the right way

> 5 gram choice at breakfast, neutrals at snack, 5 gram choice at
> lunch, neutrals at snack, 5 gram choice at dinner, 5 gram choice
> at bedtime, 5 gram choice in the middle of the night if you
> awaken.

5 gram counter carbs . . . the wrong way — this will slow fat-burning and weight loss:

> 5 gram choice at breakfast, 2 gram choice at snack, 5 gram
> choice at lunch, 3 gram choice at snack, 5 gram choice at
> dinner, 5 gram choice for night snack, 5 gram choice at bedtime,
> 5 gram choice in the middle of the night.

2. Are you undereating neutral foods?

Some people are so accustomed to eating less to lose weight faster that
they bring this mind-set to the Diabetes Miracle. At first, it may seem
counterproductive to liberally eat historically forbidden foods such as
peanut butter, pistachios, olives, cheese, and avocado. If you consistently consume fewer calories than your body requires to maintain
bodily functions, you will actually slow your metabolic rate. It may
seem counterintuitive, but eating a liberal amount of neutral foods
will promote continued weight loss.

3. Do you find yourself skipping between-meal snacks?

In an effort to lose weight, some people decide it would be in their
best interest to cut out snacks and stick to three main meals. They are
not used to eating within an hour of waking up, not letting more than
five hours pass without eating, eating a snack right before bed, or in
the middle of the night. These inclusions of meals and snacks actually
stoke your metabolic rate and help you burn fat faster.

4. Are you stuck in your exercise routine?

If day after day, month after month, you take the same exact walk at the same time for the same distance at the same pace, your body becomes used to it and doesn't respond with the desired fat burn. Consider changing the time of day you exercise, as well as the intensity, the duration, the speed, or the type of exercise you do.

If you have been doing the same exercise routine for more than three months, it's time to change it up. (For much more on exercise, see pages Chapter 12.)

5. If you began the Diabetes Miracle with very high sugar, cholesterol, triglycerides, insulin, or hemoglobin A1C, it might take a little longer than average to make a dent in your body weight because your body will always "clean house" on the inside before it burns fat on the outside.

A person who begins the Diabetes Miracle with high blood fats or blood sugar will require extra time for his body to consume the excess sugar and blood fats before it can turn its attention to burning excess body fat. Now that your labs are more normal, your weight loss will follow the expectation for your next eight-week period.

THE RULE OF DECREASING HEMOGLOBIN A1C

Remember that for every point your hemoglobin A1C decreases, a 5-pound weight gain occurs. Your body will have to burn off this fat gain before it can work on your desired weight loss.

The health benefits you derive from normal blood sugar far outweigh slower weight loss. When your blood sugar and lipids normalize, you won't be dealing with this issue. Thankfully, the Diabetes Miracle is a fat-burning program, so fat produced will be fat burned.

6. Are you taking medication that causes blood sugar to rise?
Steroid-based medications inherently cause blood sugar to rise. Examples of these medications are prednisone and cortisone; other medications that raise blood sugar can be found on page 98. If your health conditions necessitate this type of medication and your physician has your dose at the lowest effective dose for you, just know that your weight loss will naturally be slower because of this side effect. However, you will eventually lose weight.

7. Do you have other undiagnosed, untreated, or undertreated metabolic issues?
Everyone with prediabetes and type 2 diabetes begins the Diabetes Miracle with a hormonal imbalance of insulin. It's also true that at the end of Step 1, insulin levels should be in balance. If your fat loss is not in the expected range, and you ruled out all the other possibilities for what may have slowed weight loss, perhaps you have additional unresolved hormonal imbalances. If you've answered "no" to the preceding six possible causes for inadequate weight loss, ask your physician to check your thyroid panel, cortisol level, or fasting insulin level. Some underlying metabolic conditions require attention before you can get the full weight-loss benefit from this program. Don't despair because the program has already produced great benefits internally. Once the other hormonal imbalance is remedied, you won't miss a beat. Stay on the program.

I tend to get shaky, dizzy, sweaty, and anxious about forty minutes into my exercise class, bike ride, run, or anytime I exercise. I feel wiped out, my muscles burn or ache, and I'm very tired the rest of the day. What can be causing this?

Keep in mind that after Day 4 of Step 1, your liver and muscles were purposely depleted of glycogen stores to enable your pancreas and liver to rest. There is enough carbohydrate in the neutral foods of Step 1 to fuel approximately thirty minutes of normal-intensity exercise. If you exercise for thirty minutes by walking, treadmill walking, walking on the elliptical, biking, gardening, or doing yoga, you will not need to make any modifications in your diet to accommodate your exercise in Step 1. If you exercise more than thirty minutes during Step 1, you may need to "fuel forward" to prevent hypoglycemia or "hitting a wall" (muscles that ache, burn, or feel fatigued).

Step 1 "Fueling it Forward"

When your exercise will last more than thirty minutes and if you are taking no oral medications or insulin to lower blood sugar, take 15 grams of fast-acting carbohydrate to fuel the upcoming thirty minutes of activity. Fueling it forward will help to power a terrific workout that will enhance your program and leave you with plenty of energy for the rest of the day.

Examples of 15 grams of fast-acting carbs appropriate for exercise include 8 ounces Gatorade, ½ banana, ½ cup natural applesauce, three to four glucose tabs, ½ cup juice (can be diluted), 1 tablespoon honey, and 3 teaspoons of sugar dissolved in water.

Normally you would not consume these foods on Step 1. You are allowed to have them only when you are using them to fuel your upcoming exercise, which will allow your blood sugar to return back to normal after those thirty minutes.

This amount of carbohydrate will fuel the muscles for the first thirty minutes of exercise. For the next thirty minutes, you will need to take another 15 grams of carbs, and repeat the fueling for any additional thirty minutes of activity. For an hourlong spin class, for example, drink 8 ounces of Gatorade just before class, spin for thirty minutes, and drink 8 additional ounces of Gatorade before spinning for the remaining thirty minutes of class.

At the end of high-intensity exercise that lasts longer than thirty minutes, eat a good source of protein within thirty minutes after the end of the activity. Choose something like a cheese stick, low-carb protein drink, or the protein that will be contained in your next meal.

If I take medication for diabetes (oral medication or insulin), should I still fuel forward?

If you have type 2 diabetes and use oral blood glucose–lowering medication or insulin, you should test your blood sugar before your workout. If your pre-workout reading is:

- **Under 100** at the start of activity, fuel it forward as directed.
- **Between 101–180:** There is probably no need to fuel it forward at the start of activity because you may have enough circulating blood sugar to fuel the first thirty minutes. At the thirty-minute mark, begin to fuel the next thirty minutes as directed.
- **181–280:** There should be no need to fuel it forward; there is enough fuel to support your workout.
- **Over 280:** When blood sugar is this elevated, it may be better to assess the reason for the high readings before you try to lower them with exercise. Drink plenty of water, and don't exert yourself with exercise. If high readings persist, contact your doctor for possible medication intervention. An unexpectedly high blood sugar may indicate that you are sick or getting sick, have an infection, forgot your glucose-lowering medication, may be under high stress, or are experiencing high levels of pain.

This system helps prevent those who take glucose-lowering medication from becoming hypoglycemic. Remember that hypoglycemia can happen hours after a workout because exercise helps muscles to uptake glucose. If you have the symptoms of hypoglycemia, always test and treat if necessary.

Instead of fueling forward with honey, sugar, or fruit, can I use a candy bar with 15 grams of carb?

You might notice that all of the choices listed to fuel it forward are pure carbohydrate, with no protein or fat. Chocolate is a combination of carb, protein, and fat; its sugar release is a bit slower than the same amount of carbs from 4 ounces of juice. This is because the protein and fat slow the absorption of sugar. With fueling it forward, you want the sugar to rise, get burned, rise, and get burned, with no residual or leftover effects.

I have type 2 diabetes, high cholesterol/triglycerides, high blood pressure, and depression and take medication for all of these medical conditions. I read that gastric bypass surgery (weight-loss surgery) is ideal for me because I have many pounds to lose and many health conditions. Wouldn't it be easier to have a little nip/tuck and say good-bye to my diabetes and health conditions—not to mention all those expensive medications?

Every medical condition you mention, all the medications you take, and your present weight and blood sugar levels are a product of uncontrolled Met B.

Gastric bypass surgery is far more than a nip/tuck procedure. In a typical gastric bypass, your GI tract will be permanently altered in major ways: Your stomach will be completely cut, leaving you with a very small pouch (approximately 2 ounces after surgery), while the rest of the stomach is disconnected and will no longer receive food. The first part of your small intestine will be cut (this is the part that absorbs many vitamins and minerals), and the remaining intestine will be reconnected to the stomach pouch. So you are left with a very small-capacity pouch and have permanently removed the portion of your intestine that normally absorbs much high-quality nutrition. Keep in mind that your pancreas was not bypassed. It is still alive and in its Met B condition. It stands to reason that if you can only fit 2 ounces of food in your stomach, you will lose weight. In addition, you are no longer able to absorb all the nutrition from that miniscule amount of food. If you try to overeat, you will throw up any food in excess of 2 ounces. So, for about eighteen months, those with Met B who have had gastric bypass think they have found the holy grail: They are losing weight, burning fat, can't overeat or they will vomit, and can't even absorb what they do eat.

Within the first eighteen months or so after surgery, your pouch will gradually expand to hold about 1 cup of whatever you ingest. It is at this point that many people with Met B notice their weight loss cease. At close to the two-year mark, they are beginning to regain weight. This is because they can accommodate enough food to cause a rise in blood sugar and trigger insulin response. Their cravings, fatigue, poor memory, depression—all the symptoms of uncontrolled Met B— begin to return. Slowly but very assuredly, weight, cholesterol, triglycerides, blood pressure, blood sugar, and depression seep back in. I'm sure you've seen many people three years after bypass surgery beginning to morph back into the person they were before the surgery.

There is no cure for type 2 diabetes. Gastric bypass surgery is no exception—it does not cure the condition. You will be left with a permanently rewired GI tract, will forever malabsorb important nutrients, will have to take special supplements for life, and can end up exactly where you started. Ironically, I see many post–gastric bypass patients for weight regain. They all have Met B, and they all end up following the Diabetes Miracle.

So, unless your weight is causing immediate life-threatening issues that require immediate weight loss through drastic measures, think long and hard about weight-loss surgery. In the end, you will have a rewired GI tract and still need to follow a healthy diet and lifestyle to maintain your loss and control your diabetes.

Before taking any drastic measures, give the Diabetes Miracle a solid chance. It really is an eating program that is geared to your unique metabolism and will help you lose weight and inches. I've worked with many patients who were considering gastric bypass surgery who decided to try the Diabetes Miracle program, saying they would see where their weight was in six months. After seeing the amazing progress in their weight and health, they decided to stick with the program and avoid major surgery. Remember, if you have Met B, you will ultimately need the Diabetes Miracle program approximately two years postsurgery as your way of life.

Once you have completed Step 1 and have given your liver and pancreas a much-needed rest, it is time to move onto Step 2, where you will learn how to get your system to process carbohydrate more normally.

STEP 2: REPROGRAMMING YOUR METABOLISM TO HANDLE CARBOHYDRATES NORMALLY

Although Step 1 might have felt like a very low-carb diet, you were still consuming carbohydrate grams from neutral vegetables, nuts, and nut butters; creamy cheeses, such as cottage cheese; some salad dressings; soy products; and more. The Diabetes Miracle's Step 1 is not an unhealthy way of life; it is, however, more restricted than your life needs to be to keep you healthy. You may have considered staying longer than the recommended eight weeks on Step 1, but there is no real benefit to remaining longer in the lowest carb phase. At the end of eight weeks, your pancreas and liver are rested, and you have much improved blood sugar, lowered lipids (cholesterol and triglycerides), decreased insulin resistance, improved energy, and lost weight.

Whether a patient comes to me weighing 400 pounds or 150 pounds, if his Met B or diabetes is out of control, his scale weight does not determine his length of time in Step 1. Both the 400-pound and the 150-pound patient who have successfully completed Step 1 will be encouraged to move to Step 2 after eight weeks. If, however, you would like to remain longer in Step 1, feel free to do so.

On Step 2, you will reintroduce an increased amount of mild, healthy carbohydrate (the preferred fuel for your body and brain) and train your metabolism to function normally, without turning the insulin faucet back to the high setting.

Step 2 is also a weight-reduction phase and, done correctly, will allow for the same expected fat loss as was listed for Step 1 (see pages 168–170).

On the day you begin Step 2, record your starting weight and your body measurements. (See table on page 335.) You will reweigh and remeasure in eight weeks, just like you did on Step 1. Look up your expected weight loss for the upcoming eight weeks, and you are good to go.

Step 2 is a very unique part of the Diabetes Miracle program. Other lower-carb programs add carbs without direction as to the amount, type, and timing of carb reintroduction. As a result, other low-carb diets begin to unravel when carbohydrate foods return to daily intake. By following Step 2 of the Diabetes Miracle, you can continue your journey to improved blood sugar, fat loss, energy, and well-being while eating some of your favorite foods again.

YOU'LL NEVER FEAR CARBS AGAIN

After spending eight weeks on Step 1, and having experienced success with fat loss and improved blood sugar, some people become comfortable with this lower-carb lifestyle and come to view carbohydrate foods as the "bad guys." There is often a bit of fear or trepidation about moving to Step 2 because people feel they will revert to overeating and mindlessly eating carbs. They may have experienced weight regain and blood sugar spikes when reintroducing carbs on other programs and feel that this might happen on the Diabetes Miracle too.

Remember that prior to starting the Diabetes Miracle, your blood sugar and insulin had been up and down for years. You craved carbs because of overproduction of insulin. Over time, your resistance to insulin allowed excess blood sugar to remain in your blood and not enter your cells. In either case, you were hungry, and your brain signaled you to eat those carbs. Your cravings for carbs had a physical reason for being.

It wasn't the carbs that were bad, it was your pancreas's reaction to blood sugar that was out of line. Believe it or not, the right amount of carbohydrates distributed throughout the entire day (and even into the night) will help to keep you in a weight-loss mode with improved blood sugar and even more energy.

THE NEW CARB THRESHOLD: 11–20 GRAMS

During the first four days of Step 2, your liver will gradually refill with glycogen. Glycogen is stored sugar. After the fourth day, your liver will be filled and once again serve as a holding tank for glycogen. In this capacity, the liver is capable of performing one of its primary roles— self-feeding the body should more than five hours pass without eating (either during the day or at night while you sleep).

It is important to remember not to wait more than five hours without eating carbohydrates. In Step 2, when you allow more than five hours to pass, your liver will automatically self-feed the equivalent of approximately 45–65 grams of carbohydrate into the bloodstream to fuel the body over the next five hours. Your blood sugar will rise, and your Met B pancreas will strain to meet the rise in blood sugar with insulin. It is counterintuitive, but when people with diabetes wait too long to eat, they might actually see their blood sugar rise as their pancreas cannot accommodate the liver's blood sugar deposit.

If carbohydrates are reintroduced without paying attention to the amount, type, and timing, the Met B pancreas/liver combination will gradually begin to overwork again, blood sugar will rise, and any weight you have lost will return. It is the haphazard reintroduction of carbs that causes all other traditional low-carb diets to fail. When carbohydrate is reintroduced on other plans, weight regain is fast and furious, blood sugar begins to spike, and dieters think that they must forever remain on a low-carb phase to have normal blood sugar, lose weight, and keep it off. *The Diabetes Miracle* solves that problem because it systematically reintroduces the right kind of carbohydrate in the right amount and at the right time.

As you know, there are two sources of blood sugar: blood sugar derived from carbohydrate foods and that from liver release of glycogen. In Step 2, the liver is back in business and refilled with glycogen.

REINTRODUCING HIGH-CARBOHYDRATE FOODS WITHOUT TRIGGERING THE LIVER'S SELF-FEED MODE

The amount of mild carb necessary during Step 2 is the amount of carb grams that is low enough to allow the pancreas to remain relaxed but just high enough to prevent the liver from engaging in the self-feed mode. After much research in my nutrition therapy practice, I found the magic number in Step 2 to be 11–20 grams of net carbohydrate. To determine the carbohydrate grams of a food, you will use the

same formula that you used in Step 1: total carbohydrate grams –
dietary fiber = 11–20 grams net carbs.

If you regulate your carb intake throughout the day and into the
night, keeping the carbs at each interval in an amount that is neither
too much nor too little (11–20 grams total net carbs), and if the type of
carbohydrate is lower-impact and doesn't overstimulate the reawak-
ened pancreas, you will be in control of your blood sugar and
weight . . . permanently.*

THE ELEVEN RULES OF STEP 2

(These rules are similar to the rules of Step 1. See page 134.)

1. All neutral foods in Step 1 remain neutral in Step 2.
2. Eat within one hour of awakening, within one hour of going to
   sleep, and go no longer than five hours without eating
   throughout the day.
3. Drink a minimum of 64 ounces of water and decaffeinated fluid.
   (If you are 5' 3" or less, drink a minimum 48 ounces of
   water/day.)
4. Add 11–20 gram carb choices as directed to any neutral foods at
   your breakfast, lunch, dinner, bedtime, in the middle of the
   night (if you are awake), and in between any meals that exceed
   five hours. **In Step 2, the 11–20 gram carb choices are
   mandatory, not options**.
5. Use neutral foods to satisfy hunger once you've met your 11–20
   gram carb choice at meals and snacks. You may always have
   neutral foods.

---

*During the first four days of Step 2, as the liver refills with glycogen, some people no-
tice a slight bloating or feeling of fullness. This is not fat regain. A small amount of fluid
retention goes along with the process, and by the fifth day, this bloating will subside.

6. You should continue to take vitamins, minerals, and other supplements.
7. Drink green tea using a minimum of two green tea bags per day.
8. Exercise a minimum of thirty minutes, five times per week, above your normal activity. Change it up for variety.
9. If you choose to exercise in the morning before breakfast, eat an 11–20 gram carb choice before your morning workout and also at your breakfast after exercise.
10. When you go more than five hours between meals, you'll need an additional 11–20 gram carb choice at the snack between the meals. Don't remove the 11–20 gram carb choice from the next meal.
11. There is typically no need to "fuel it forward" for exercise that exceeds thirty minutes during Step 2 because your liver and muscles are once again filled with glycogen.

WHEN TO TEST YOUR BLOOD SUGAR

Testing times for those with diabetes treated with diet and exercise or diet, exercise, and oral medication:

1. First thing in the morning when you get up for the day (my typical target = 70–120 mg/dL)
2. Two hours after the start of any meal (my typical target = 140 mg/dL or less).

Testing times for those with type 2 diabetes treated with insulin:

1. Most physicians will recommend testing before breakfast, lunch, dinner, and bedtime (ideal is often 80–110, but your physician should inform you of your pre-meal goals)
2. Before/after exercise
3. If you are experiencing the symptoms of hypoglycemia.

WHEN TO EAT THE 11–20 GRAM CARB CHOICES

You will have mandatory carb placement of 11–20 grams net carbs at breakfast, lunch, dinner, bedtime, and in the middle of the night (if you are awake). If any meal occurs more than five hours after the previous meal, eat an additional 11–20 gram carb choice between the meals to keep the liver suppressed. Maintain normal blood sugar by not having too much sugar produced by your food or too little, which would cause the liver to release glycogen stores,

Here's what a typical day looks like on Step 2 on diet and exercise or diet, exercise, and oral medications:

7:00 AM   Wake up, check and log blood sugar

8:00 AM   Breakfast (requires 11–20 gram carb choice)

11:00 AM   Snack (because the time between breakfast and lunch is greater than five hours, this snack will include an 11–20 gram carb choice).

1:30 PM   Lunch: (requires 11–20 gram carb choice)

4:30 PM   Snack (because the time between lunch and dinner is greater than five hours, this snack will include 11–20 gram carb choice)

7:00 PM   Dinner (requires 11–20 gram carb choice)

9:00 PM   Check and log blood sugar

11:00 PM   Bedtime (requires 11–20 gram carb choice)

3:00 AM   I'm awake, so I'll eat an 11–20 gram carb choice.

On this day, 11–20 gram carb choices made an appearance seven times based on the day's events and timing of meals.

Here's how another day of the same week but with different timing of meals and exercise looks:

7:00 AM   Wake up, check and log blood sugar. It was 127, and I decided to exercise first thing in the morning

7:30 AM   Pre-exercise (requires 11–20 gram carb choice) as I am exercising before my first meal.

9:00 AM   Breakfast (requires 11–20 gram carb choice)

11:00 AM   Snack (neutral foods, such as nuts or cheese, if I'm hungry because breakfast and lunch occur within five hours today)

1:00 PM   Lunch (requires 11–20 gram carb choice)

3:00 PM   Check and log blood sugar

4:00 PM   Snack (Neutral foods if I'm hungry because lunch and dinner occur within five hours today)

5:30 PM   Dinner (requires 11–20 gram carb choice)

10:00 PM   Bedtime (requires 11–20 gram carb choice)

No nighttime snack because I slept through the night.

On this day, 11–20 gram carb choices made an appearance five times based on the day's events and timing of meals.

As you can see, your carb placement may change on a daily basis, just as your life does. You don't have to modify your life to fit Step 2; you will modify Step 2 to fit your life.

CHOOSING THE RIGHT TYPE OF CARBS FOR STEP 2

Choosing your carbs wisely is the key to success in Step 2. Although you can get 16 grams of carbs from a glass of juice, the speed at which your blood sugar would respond to that pure sugar would trigger your rested pancreas—potentially undoing the benefits you gained in Step 1.

The carbohydrate suggestions for Step 2 are lower–glycemic index and lower–glycemic load. What makes Step 2 different from any other carb reintroduction is that it takes into account glycemic index, glycemic load, amount of net carb grams, and timing of net carb grams.

Notice that for the most part, the higher the fiber grams in a food choice, the lower-impact the carb. You'll also notice some healthy substitutes for some old favorites: Suggested breads will be whole grain,* rice should be brown or wild rice, pasta should be whole grain or whole wheat, potatoes should be sweet potatoes rather than white, and most fruits are fresh and unprocessed. These lower-impact carbs allow for a gradual rise in blood sugar throughout the entire day, which will enable normal insulin flow throughout the day. Step 2 allows you to awaken your carbohydrate metabolism in a predetermined way to cause smooth blood sugar curves rather than steep peaks and low valleys.*

THE PERFECT GENTLE CARB CHOICE

Crunchy Herbed Whole-Grain Crackers:
Serving size: 12 crackers
Total carbs: 19 grams
Dietary fiber: 5 grams

19–5 = 14 net carb grams. With net carbs between 11–20 grams and fiber well over 2 grams, this is a perfect choice.

NOT A GREAT GENTLE CARB CHOICE

Crunchy Herbed Crackers:
Serving size: 12 crackers
Total carbs: 14 grams
Dietary fiber: 0 grams

---

*Check labels of bread, rolls, English muffins, bread products, wraps, cereal, crackers, bars, and other grain-based foods to make sure that the dietary fiber on the nutrient facts label is 2 grams or more.

14–0= 14 net carb grams. Although it fits the 11–20 grams net carb, these crackers have zero fiber. It would not be a low-impact carb choice but would instead act as a wild carb and turn into blood sugar at a fast rate. These fiber-free crackers are not a good choice for Step 2.

WEIGHT LOSS AND STEP 2

As in Step 1, it is best not to weigh yourself until after eight weeks of Step 2. The Diabetes Miracle is a hormone-balancing program. When you reintroduce carbohydrates to your metabolism in Step 2, your body has to hormonally adjust to the mild rise in blood sugar. Simply follow the program as directed, weigh and measure yourself at the beginning and the end of the eight weeks, and your results will fall within the expected range. You will lose weight, and it will be fat loss. Your pounds lost and inches lost should match each other.

After the first few days of Step 2, your blood sugar will normalize. If, after a week on Step 2, your readings are out of range and you know you are following the Step 2 guidelines correctly and exercising as directed, you should consider contacting your physician because medication might be in order.

STEP 2 FOOD LISTS

The following list includes excellent gentle, lower-impact carb choices. Choose any food from the lower-impact carbs list for your breakfast, lunch, dinner, bedtime snack, and in the middle of the night if you are awake. If time between meals exceeds five hours, place an extra carb serving between them.

All portions shown are ready to eat and equal 11–20 grams of carb.

BREADS*

2 slices thin-sliced, light whole-grain bread
1 slice whole-grain bread
1 light whole-grain English muffin
½ whole-grain English muffin
1 light or lower-carb whole-grain pita
½ whole-grain pita.

CEREALS AND GRAINS

½ cup cooked oatmeal
½ cup cooked barley
½ cup of cooked brown or wild rice
½ cup of cooked whole-grain pasta (cook al dente)
½ cup cooked bulgur
½ cup cooked quinoa
Dry cereal (11–20 grams carbs and 2 grams or more fiber).

CRACKERS, POPCORN, PRETZELS, AND CHIPS

The foods listed below should contain 11–20 grams of carbs and 2
grams or more of fiber.

Crackers, whole grain
3 cups popcorn (light or hot air preferred—popped without
    partially hydrogenated oils)
Whole-grain pretzels
Tortilla chips (baked preferred).

---

*Read the label for bread, cereal, bars, and crackers to make certain that dietary fiber
is 2 grams or greater.

PROTEIN OR CEREAL BARS

Any protein bars you eat should have 11–20 grams net carbs and 2 grams of fiber or more.

VEGETABLES AND LEGUMES

½ cup corn

½ ear fresh corn

½ cup peas

½ cup legumes, such as kidney beans, lentils, lima beans, chick-peas, white beans, black beans, and white kidney beans

½ whole or ½ cup mashed sweet potato or yam

1 ½ cups cooked carrots

1 cup beets.

SOUPS

Canned or prepared soups should be the proper portion size and provide 11–20 grams carb and 2 grams or more fiber

1 cup tomato soup (water-based)

½ cup lentil soup (or check label)

½ cup split pea soup (or check label).

1 cup meat chili with beans

FRUIT

Whole fruit choices should be average in size. Consider a serving of fruit to contain 15 grams of net carbs. Because of this, you may have a serving of fruit and a 5 gram counter at the same meal or snack on Step 2.

1 apple

1 pear

1 peach

2 plums

1 nectarine

12 cherries

½ cup natural applesauce

½ grapefruit (not recommended if you are taking the medication
Lipitor)

1 cup whole strawberries (approximately 6–8 berries)

¾ cup blackberries

¾ cup blueberries

1 cup raspberries

2 clementine oranges or 2 small tangerines

8 dried apricot halves or 4 fresh apricots

12 grapes

1 orange

¾ cup pineapple cubes

½ banana

1 cup melon (honeydew, watermelon, canteloupe).

MILK AND DAIRY

The following should have 11–20 grams net carb.

8 fluid ounces or 1 cup milk (fat-free, nonfat, 1 percent, 2 percent)

¾ cup plain yogurt or Greek yogurt

8 fluid ounces or 1 cup buttermilk

Fruit-flavored yogurt with nonnutritive sweetener

½ cup sugar-free or fat-free pudding

No-sugar-added ice cream products.

SAMPLE MENUS FOR STEP 2

BREAKFAST

Egg muffin sandwich: Light multigrain English muffin (11–20
grams net carb, 2 grams fiber or more)

(continued)

Poached egg

1 slice of Canadian bacon and 1 slice of low-fat cheese

Coffee with light creamer

1 slice of light whole-wheat bread (5 grams of net carb) spread with
    Natural peanut butter and ½ banana sliced (15 grams net carbs)

Cold glass of almond milk

Low-carb protein shake (2 grams net carb)

Sliced apple with natural peanut butter (15 grams net carbs)

Green tea with lemon

French toast: Dip 2 slices light multigrain bread in beaten egg and
    brown on both sides in a hot skillet that was sprayed with olive
    oil cooking spray. (11–20 grams net carb, 2 grams or more fiber)

Top with whipped cream and a dollop of carb-free jelly

Decaf coffee with cream and stevia

6–8 sliced strawberries over low-fat cottage cheese or part-skim
    ricotta cheese (11–20 grams carb)

Sprinkle with a handful of chopped walnuts

Green tea with lemon

Thinly sliced smoked salmon (lox)

Low-carb mini-bagel (11–20 grams net carb, 2 or more grams fiber)

Whipped cream cheese

Green tea with lemon

½ cup cooked oatmeal sprinkled with cinnamon and chopped
    walnuts (11–20 grams net carb, 2 or more grams fiber)

1 cup organic unsweetened almond milk

Coffee with light cream and stevia

LUNCH

Dip of cottage cheese with tomato slices
Low-carb mini-bagel (11–20 grams net carb, 2 or more grams fiber)
Whipped butter
Sparkling water with lemon slice

Sliced, oven-baked turkey breast
Lettuce and sliced tomatoes
2 slices light multigrain bread (11–20 grams net carb, 2 or more
    grams fiber)
Cheesy chips (see page 158)
Sugar-free drink

Sliced, baked ham and low-fat cheese
1 sandwich thin (11–20 grams net carb, 2 or more grams fiber)
Lettuce and tomato slices
Light mayo or small amount of regular mayo or mustard
Herbal iced tea with stevia

Shrimp, tuna, or chicken salad on a bed of romaine lettuce
Tomato wedges
12 whole-grain cracker crisps (11–20 grams net carb, 2 or more
    grams fiber)
Ice water with lemon wedge

1 cup tomato soup (11–20 grams net carb)
Garden salad with olives and fresh mozzarella
Balsamic vinaigrette
Sugar-free beverage

Veggie burger (containing 5 grams or less net carbs) on a low-carb
burger bun (11–20 grams net carb, 2 or more grams fiber)
Lettuce, sliced tomato, and onions
Low-carb ketchup
Cheesy chips
Lemon water

Low-carb protein bar (11–20 grams net carb, 2 or more grams
fiber)
Bottle of water

Low-carb protein shake (5 gram counter)
Choose one: apple, peach, pear, or orange (15 grams net carb)
Handful of almonds

Grilled pork, chicken, London broil cut in cubes and stuffed into a
low-carb pita along with shredded lettuce, chopped tomatoes,
light sour cream (pita with 11–20 grams net carb, 2 or more
grams fiber)
Sugar-free beverage

DINNER

Chicken cutlets "breaded" with parmesan cheese (instead of using
bread crumbs to coat your chicken cutlets, replace with grated
parmesan cheese)
½ baked sweet potato (11–20 grams net carb)
Garden green beans
Chocolaty ricotta dessert (in ½ cup of part-skim ricotta cheese, add
½ tsp carb-free chocolate syrup, ½ packet sucralose, and ¼ tsp
vanilla. Stir and serve chilled)
Iced tea with stevia and lemon

Light beer

Barbeque chicken (use carb-free BBQ sauce)

½ ear of corn (11–20 grams net carb)

Veggie platter of raw broccoli, carrots, celery, mushrooms, and light
French onion dip

Sugar-free gelatin with light whipped topping

"Breakfast for Dinner"

Scrambled eggs with baby spinach and shredded light cheddar
cheese

Low-carb bagel (11–20 grams net carb, 2 or more grams fiber)

Whipped cream cheese

Decaffeinated coffee with creamer

Glass of white wine

Grilled salmon

½ cup brown rice (11–20 grams net carb)

Steamed spinach

Tea with stevia

Broiled flounder

½ cup lightly buttered whole-wheat pasta with parmesan cheese
and chopped fresh parsley (11–20 grams net carb, 2 or more
grams fiber)

Steamed spring vegetables

Sugar-free gelatin with whipped cream

Water with lime

5 ounces red wine

Baked beef tenderloin

½ sweet potato (11–20 grams net carb)

Steamed broccoli with lemon

Vanilla ricotta dessert (in ½ cup part of skim ricotta cheese, add ½
    tsp of vanilla and ½ packet sucralose. Stir and serve chilled)

Cubed tofu sautéed with olive oil and neutral veggies
Serve over ½ cup whole grain pasta and sprinkled with grated
    cheese (11–20 grams net carb, 2 or more grams fiber)
Garden salad with balsamic vinaigrette
Flavored seltzer water

Thinly sliced flank steak with au jus
½ cup brown rice pilaf (11–20 grams net carb)
Tender baby spinach
Green tea with lemon wedge

Baked ham
½ sweet potato (11–20 grams net carb)
Brussels sprouts
Lemony ricotta dessert with whipped cream (½ cup of part-skim
    ricotta, ¼ tsp lemon extract, ½ packet of sucralose. Stir and
    serve chilled.)

11–20 GRAM SNACKS

When an 11–20 gram snack is required, for bread and bread products,
be sure to check for 2 grams of fiber and to eat the proper portion.

Whole-grain crackers
Piece of fresh fruit from allowed list (see page 192)
1 cup nonfat or low-fat milk
Yogurt
3 cups popcorn (light or air popped preferred)
Tortilla chips (baked preferred)
Baked soy crisps
½ cup natural applesauce

Whole-wheat pretzels
Sugar-free ice cream
Sugar-free pudding
Whole-grain cereal with unsweetened soy or almond milk
Cereal bars

FREQUENTLY ASKED QUESTIONS FOR STEP 2

If I eat carb portions that are closer to 11 grams rather than 20 grams in Step 2, I'll lose weight faster, right?

The lower end of the 11–20 gram carb range offers no benefit. There is no difference in terms of weight loss, blood sugar control, or insulin rise if, on average, you choose your lower-impact carbohydrates from anywhere within the 11–20 gram range (inclusive). If, however, you are a person who uses insulin and notice that when you use a 20 gram carb choice you get a higher pre-meal glucose reading at the following meal, you may want to experiment with an 11–15 gram selection to see if you note an appreciable improvement.

During the first five days or so of Step 1, I remember that my blood sugar was erratic. Will I experience erratic blood sugar during the first days of Step 2?

During the first five days of Step 2, your liver and muscles are refilling with glycogen. I often tell my patients not to rely too much on their readings during their initial four to five days in Steps 1 or 2.

You may notice that your post-meal readings are slightly higher than they were in Step 1 because you now have 11–20 grams of appreciable carbs at a meal. You may have gotten used to two-hour post-meal readings of 95 or 101 on Step 1. It would be plausible that a normal post-meal reading on Step 2 would be 130. This is not a bad reading: blood sugar of 140 or less two hours after the start of a meal is considered to be normal.

Remember that if you skip a necessary 11–20 gram carb, your liver will intervene and release glycogen stores that would actually make your blood sugar rise higher than if you ate the 11–20 gram carb choice. Skipping these snacks between meals that are more than five hours apart can cause a rise in blood sugar.

If you skip your 11–20 gram snack before bedtime, your fasting blood sugar reading will most likely be higher because your liver will be more engaged while you sleep. Also, the later you sleep in the morning, the higher your blood sugar will rise. Blood sugar checked at 6:00 AM will be lower than blood sugar checked at 9:00 AM if there was no food from the night before.

If your blood sugar rises out of target range while on any step of the Diabetes Miracle program, and you are certain that you are eating and exercising as prescribed, contact your physician because you may require medication.

When I wake up in the morning, I'm perfectly content to eat a low-carb shake (mine has just 3 grams of net carbs). I can't imagine taking an 11–20 gram carb choice when I am not even hungry and don't want those extra calories and carb grams.

If you skip the required carbs while you are on Steps 2 or 3, your liver will release approximately 45–65 grams of carbohydrate, which is undoubtedly more sugar than you would consider eating and could actually cause your blood sugar to rise. The 11–20 gram carb choices are not options; they are mandatory and necessary. In fact, they enable you to lose weight and keep blood sugar regular. Be sure to follow the timed 11–20 gram carbohydrate schedule.

If you are not hungry at a particular meal, instead of skipping the carb, you can have a smaller portion of heart-healthy protein and fat.

My blood sugar is normal when I wake up in the morning, but when I check two hours after the start of a meal, it often exceeds 140. What could be causing the increase?

Your fasting blood sugar is composed of sugar that is self-fed from the liver's glycogen stores while you are asleep. Testing your blood sugar two hours after the start of a meal is checking how your body is handling the blood sugar produced by the meal you just ate.

The following is a quick checklist for determining why a post-meal reading might be elevated:*

- Did you consume the correct amount and type of carb at the meal in question?
- Did you take your additional 11–20 grams net carbs snack before the meal if it was necessary?
- Were all the other foods you ate neutral?
- If you require diabetes medication, did you take it that day?
- Did you exercise with regularity this week?
- Are you getting sick?*
- Are you in pain?*
- Are you under a higher than usual amount of stress?*

If and when everything's in order and your numbers remain elevated, it may be time to discuss medication with your doctor. Remember that medication need not be permanent. When the pain, illness, or stress passes, you may no longer require the diabetes medication.

---

*Sometimes it's something other than food that can be affecting your readings.

I have had type 2 diabetes for twenty years. Before I found out about the Diabetes Miracle, I followed a traditional diabetes diet and eventually required two diabetes medications: metformin and glimiperide. In the past, even with the medications at increased doses, my blood sugar was never in the normal zone. Now that I'm on the Diabetes Miracle plan, I have actually experienced hypoglycemia at least three times in the past week. Should I stop taking the medication?

This is an excellent illustration of why self-monitoring your blood sugar is so important. First, call your doctor and report the hypoglycemia. She should ask the time of day you experienced the low blood sugar, what you ate prior to the event, if you exercised before your sugar dropped, and what the actual readings were.

Your home monitoring numbers will provide your physician with information to help decide which medication to decrease, which to leave as is, and eventually which to eliminate. With your help, your doctor can quickly make the right medication decisions. Never stop taking a medication without first checking with your physician.

I'm afraid to add carbohydrates back into my diet. I have diabetes, and I'm sure my blood sugar will fly out of control with the return of carbohydrates. Should I just live in Step 1?

There is no reason to fear reintroducing carbohydrates into your diet. The Diabetes Miracle adds carbohydrates in a very methodical, proven way with three factors in place:

A *set amount of carb grams*: 11–20 grams net carbs at meals and some snacks (low glycemic load).

Lower-impact carbs are recommended to ease the pancreas into releasing insulin (low glycemic index).

A recommended timing schedule for carbohydrate inclusion that helps to keep blood sugar smooth and prevents the liver from rocking the boat with unnecessary glycogen release.

Because of the very methodical introduction of carbs, you should not expect to see a large swing in blood sugar readings. Prior to beginning Step 1, you suffered through blood sugar peaks and valleys caused by eating too many carb grams at some meals; skipping carbs at other meals; taking inadequate carbs to suppress the liver; having long gaps between meals; consuming high–glycemic index carbs like white pasta, rice, chips, candy, and cookies on a regular basis; and possibly not taking regular exercise.

Step 2 stresses the appropriate amount of carb grams at meals and snacks, all of which will be of lower–glycemic index. You will continue to be encouraged to regularly exercise, drink adequate water/decaf liquids, and try to lessen stress. This is a much different scenario from your lifestyle prior to beginning the Diabetes Miracle.

How can you be certain that you are tolerating the reintroduction of carbs? Self-monitor your blood sugar on a daily basis, and after eight weeks, reweigh and remeasure to assess weight loss and inches lost. Repeat lab work to ascertain positive lab changes.*

SLIP-UP REMEDIES

What if I slip-up on Step 2? I have a class reunion to attend next month and a business trip to Paris this summer. I want to stay on the plan, but I'm pretty certain I'll have more than two slip-ups in a week during those two weeks.

---

*Please note that in the first four days of Step 2, your liver and muscles are refilling with glycogen stores. Your blood sugar readings may appear erratic during the first four to five days until sugar stores are refilled. After Day 4 of Step 2, your readings should fall into a definite pattern.

Slip-ups occur when you do not eat carbs of the right type in the right amount or at the right time. Some slip-ups include:

- More than 20 grams net carbs at a meal or snack
- Less than 11 grams net carbs at a meal or snack
- Skipping your 11–20 gram bedtime carb target
- Skipping your 11–20 gram target within an hour of waking up
- Going more than five hours without an 11–20 carb target between meals.

How frequently you slip up determines what you need to do to remedy the situation.

The one-meal slip-up occurs when you attend a dinner with friends, a celebration meal, or a single holiday meal; or when find yourself in need of a "one-meal break" after being on the program for a period of time.

Unlike other diet plans that encourage you to save up your points or calories to use for a special meal, people with Met B, prediabetes, or type 2 diabetes cannot save 11–20 gram carb targets and lump them into one pile. Each missed 11–20 gram carb choice would cause the liver to self-feed, blood sugar to spike, the pancreas to try to release insulin, and your body to gain fat. If you are on blood sugar–lowering medication, missing your 11–20 gram carb target at a meal or necessary snack could lead to hypoglycemia. Adding all the saved carb into one meal will cause an overdose of carbs and resultant high blood sugar, increased pancreas involvement, and weight gain.

The beauty of the Diabetes Miracle is that if you find yourself "off program" for a meal, you can do nothing to make up for it. Take all your necessary 11–20 gram carb targets in the day leading up to the meal, and remember to resume your 11–20 gram carb targets after the meal. That's it. Just be sure to get right back on the program afterward.

Those with diabetes will find their blood sugar will rise after a meal that is off the program, but this blip should not extend more than five hours after the mistake. You cannot skip the next 11–20 gram to make up for this because without this carb choice, your blood sugar would rise higher from the liver release. Just get right back into the Step 2 saddle, and you will be fine.

Extended slip-ups occur during a vacation, long weekend, or holiday period. If you find yourself having more than two slip-ups in a one-week period, you must return to Step 1 for ten days to clean up the metabolic mess. If you are going on vacation, stay on Step 2 as closely as possible, but if you slip up more than twice during that week, just resign yourself to clean up when you get back.

When more than two slip-ups occur in a week, do what I call the "big eraser." Commit yourself to doing ten days of Step 1. After the ten-day clean-up, you will return to Step 2, and your weight, blood sugar, and energy will be back to normal again.

What else could make me return to Step 1 for a clean-up?

Aside from dietary slip-ups, high stress affects your ability to control blood sugar. Everyone has normal stress in his life — job, family demands, finances — but more intense stress, such as a death in the family, divorce, car accident, surgery, or painful injury, can cause your body to release stress hormones which, in turn, cause blood sugar to rise. If you find yourself in a period of high stress, the safest place to be is Step 1. On Step 1, your liver and muscles are emptied of glycogen stores, and you are not consuming high-impact carbs. Your pancreas and liver will rest, and your blood sugar, weight, health, and cravings will not suffer.

It takes four days to empty liver glycogen stores on Step 1, but once glycogen is depleted, the rise in stress hormones — such as adrenaline epinephrine, and cortisol—cannot cause the liver to react with wild sugar release.

If you forget to revert to Step 1 during a high-stress time period, once you get your bearings, return to Step 1 for a ten-day period for every week of your high stress.

Just as high stress can cause your metabolism to become over-wrought, so can pain and illness. If you experience a period of pain that lasts three days or more (throw your back out, sprain an ankle, have a migraine headache or a toothache), you will need a ten-day period of Step 1 after the pain subsides to reset the pancreas/liver combination. If you have been under stress, in pain, or ill for a period of more than two weeks, or if you have been "off program" for more than two weeks, you will require more than ten days of Step 1 to get back on course. If you've been off the program for two weeks or more, consider a month or more of Step 1.

To recap, if you are off the program for one meal, it's no problem; continue on Step 2. You are allowed two mistakes per week. If you are off the program for three days to two weeks or less, you will need to do ten days of Step 1. If you are off program for two weeks or more, you will need to do a minimum of four weeks of Step 1.

Do I still need to fuel it forward when I exercise for more than thirty minutes on Step 2?

In Step 2, your liver and muscles have regained their stores of glycogen. If you have prediabetes or type 2 diabetes and take no blood sugar–lowering medication, you will not be required to fuel it forward for exercise that will last up to sixty minutes. If you intend to exercise for periods of longer than sixty minutes, you should fuel it forward for upcoming thirty-minute blocks of exercise in excess of one hour.

For example: Lunch at 1:00 PM; exercise begins at 2:30 PM. You are in Step 2, and your muscles and liver have glycogen stores. Your lunch began at 1:00 PM, so you know that you must have your next 11–20 gram choice before 6:00 PM. You are planning to have dinner about 7:00 PM and will begin to exercise at 2:30 PM. As long as you are finished exercising by 3:30, you will not need to fuel it forward. You can take your 11–20 gram snack (as well as some protein) when you are through with exercise. If you are going to exercise longer than one hour, you will need to take a quick fuel source (eight ounces of Gatorade, ½ banana, three to four glucose tablets, or 1 tablespoon honey) at 3:30 PM for the upcoming half hour of exercise.

1:00 PM	Lunch
2:30 PM	Exercise begins
3:30 PM	Take 11–20 gram carb choice because exercise is exceeding sixty minutes
4:00 PM	Exercise is over. Take 11–20 gram carb snack and some protein within the next half hour
7:00 PM	Dinner.

If you have type 2 diabetes, it's a great idea to begin exercise one to one and a half hours after a meal or a snack. Post-meal blood sugar is highest one to two hours after eating. Exercise after eating will automatically lower your blood sugar and has a glucose-lowering effect for hours afterward. Exercising after eating also greatly lowers the risk of hypoglycemia.

If I have type 2 diabetes and take medication for diabetes (use oral blood glucose–lowering medication or insulin), should I test my blood sugar before I workout to decide how to proceed?

Yes, those who take meds or insulin should test before exercising. If your pre-workout reading is:

- **Under 100** at the start of activity, fuel it forward as directed.
- **Between 101–180:** There is probably no need to fuel it forward at the start of activity because you may have enough circulating blood sugar to fuel the first thirty minutes. At the thirty-minute mark, begin to fuel the next thirty as directed.
- **181–280:** There should be no need to fuel it forward; there is enough fuel to support your workout of up to sixty minutes.
- **Over 280:** When blood sugar is this elevated, it may be better to assess the reason for the high readings before you try to lower them with exercise. Drink plenty of water, and don't exert yourself with exercise. If high readings persist, contact your doctor for possible medication intervention. An unexpectedly high blood sugar may indicate that you are sick or getting sick, have an infection, forgot your glucose-lowering medication, may be under high stress, or are experiencing high levels of pain.

Once you have successfully reset your liver and pancreas (with a minimum of eight weeks of Step 1) and learned how to control carb intake to keep blood sugar levels in check, have normal Met B–related lab work on as little medication as possible, and like the way you look and feel, (with a minimum of eight weeks of Step 2), you are ready to move on to Step 3!

STEP 3: MAINTAINING GREAT HEALTH FOR A LIFETIME

WHAT TO EXPECT IN STEP 3

- **How long will I stay in Step 3?** Step 3 is the maintenance phase of the Diabetes Miracle. In fact, it is more of a way of life than a step of a diet. So, rather than thinking of it as a step that comes to an end, think of it as the beginning of the rest of a healthy life.

- **What is the purpose of Step 3?** Step 1 enabled you to rest and rehabilitate your overwrought metabolism. Step 2 helped you to reprogram your metabolism to accept and process carbohydrates in a normal way as it reset your metabolism and normalized your blood sugar. Step 3 establishes your own personal carbohydrate range, which allows you to enjoy great blood sugar and overall health while keeping you energized and at your desired weight permanently. The good news? Step 3 contains a greater quantity and variety of carbohydrate foods.

- **How will I feel on Step 3?** Step 3 allows you to choose, on any given day at any meal, the amount of carbohydrate you would like to consume within your personal recommended range. You may enjoy more grams of carbohydrates as well as a greater variety of carbohydrate choices. Life is good, and you are going to feel great.

A SLIGHT CHANGE IN TERMINOLOGY: CHANGING "CARB GRAMS" INTO "CARB SERVINGS"

In Step 3, you will easily calculate the number of carbohydrate servings that match your individual needs. In Step 2, 11–20 grams net carbs were mandatory at breakfast, lunch, dinner, bedtime, in the middle of the night (if you were awake), and between any meals that were more than five hours apart. In Step 3, these 11–20 gram amounts will be referred to as "carb servings," and you will discover just how many of these servings your body can handle to maintain your desired weight and health.

CONSIDER 15 GRAMS OF NET CARBS TO BE ONE CARB SERVING

Because the range for a carb serving is between 11–20 grams net carbs, 15 grams of carbohydrate—the midpoint between the numbers 11 and 20—equals one carb serving here. Using 15 grams of net carbs makes reading food labels convenient for Step 3. You will use the same net carb formula that you used in Steps 1 and 2 to determine the number of carb servings that are in a portion of any packaged item. Total carbohydrate grams – dietary fiber grams = net carb grams. The twist? If you divide your net carb grams by 15, you can find the number of carb servings in any food. For example:

Theresa's whole-grain panini
Serving size: 1 panini
Total carbohydrate grams = 48 grams
Dietary fiber grams = 3 grams
48 – 3 = 45 total net carbs
45 ÷ 15 = 3 carb servings

Ramesh's brown rice and lentils
Serving size: 1 cup
Total carbohydrate grams: 33 grams
Dietary fiber grams: 2 grams
33 – 2 = 31 total net carbs
31 ÷ 15 = 2 carb servings

For those who are not fond of math, this chart will show you the conversion of net carb grams into carb servings.

If your net carb grams are	*Your carb servings are*
5.5–10 gram range	½ carb serving
11–20 gram range	1 carb serving
21–25 gram range	1½ carb servings
26–35 gram range	2 carb servings
36–40 gram range	2½ carb servings
41–50 gram range	3 carb servings
51–55 gram range	3 ½ carb servings
56–65 gram range	4 carb servings

HOW MANY CARB SERVINGS CAN YOU HAVE?

Now that you have achieved your desired weight, have normal blood sugar on little to no medication, have seen marked improvements in your labs, have been able to decrease medications with doctor approval, and look and feel great, it's time to maintain the new and improved you. How do you know how many carb servings you can maximally have per day and still maintain all of your great results? Your carb range will vary based on your gender, age, and activity level (over and above your typical day's activities). Use these guidelines to assess your activity level:

- Sedentary: thirty minutes or less of physical activity four to five times per week
- Moderate: thirty to sixty minutes of moderate physical activity four to five times per week
- High: more than one hour of moderate to intense physical activity, four to five times per week.

Based on your gender, age, and activity level, the Carb Charts beginning on page 213 will help you ascertain the maximum number of carbohydrate servings you can use per day.

THE RULES FOR STEP 3

The object of Step 3 is to know your personal carb range and spread your carb servings throughout your day the way you like them. Every day can be different, and there are only a few guidelines to follow to keep your program on the up and up.

Remember that too many carb grams at one time will overwork the pancreas, and too few carb grams at one time will allow your liver to engage. The carb-spreading rules are similar to those in Step 2, with two additions.

1. You must start your day with a minimum of 1 carb serving (11–20 grams) within one hour of wake-up.
2. You must end your day with a minimum of 1 carb serving (11–20 grams) within one hour of sleep.
3. You must put an additional carb serving (11–20 grams) between your meals if they are separated by more than five hours.
4. If you are awake in the middle of the night, you can have a one carb serving as a snack. (This is in addition to your carb allotment for the day.)

5. If you exercise first thing in the morning before breakfast, you must have one carb serving (11–20 grams) prior to the workout.

6. You cannot exceed four carb servings (56–65 grams of carbs total) at any one time (assuming your carb allotment allows it—see chart on pages 213–218).

7. You must use a minimum of one carb serving (11–20 grams) at a meal or necessary snack.

WOMEN

CARB CHART

Female 5'0" to 5'3" with a maintenance weight of 100–130 pounds

Age	Activity	Maximum carb servings/day
Teens–age 20	Sedentary	8.5
	Moderate	9
	High	9.5
20s and 30s	Sedentary	8
	Moderate	8.5
	High	9
40s and 50s	Sedentary	7.5
	Moderate	8
	High	8.5
60s and 70s	Sedentary	7
	Moderate	7.5
	High	8
Over 80	Sedentary	6.5
	Moderate	7
	High	7.5

Age	Activity	Maximum carb servings/day

Female 5'4" to 5'7" with a maintenance weight of 120–150 pounds

Age	Activity	Maximum carb servings/day
Teens–age 20	Sedentary	9.5
	Moderate	10
	High	10.5
20s and 30s	Sedentary	9
	Moderate	9.5
	High	10
40s and 50s	Sedentary	8.5
	Moderate	9
	High	9.5
60s and 70s	Sedentary	8
	Moderate	8.5
	High	9
Over 80	Sedentary	7.5
	Moderate	8
	High	8.5

Female 5'8" to 5'11" with a maintenance weight of 140–170 pounds

Age	Activity	Maximum carb servings/day
Teens–age 20	Sedentary	10
	Moderate	11
	High	12
20s and 30s	Sedentary	9.5
	Moderate	10.5
	High	11.5
40s and 50s	Sedentary	9
	Moderate	10
	High	11
60s and 70s	Sedentary	8.5
	Moderate	9.5
	High	10.5
Over 80	Sedentary	8
	Moderate	9
	High	10

Age	Activity	Maximum carb servings/day

Female 6'0" to 6'3" with a maintenance weight of 155–185 pounds

Age	Activity	Maximum carb servings/day
Teens–age 20	Sedentary	11
	Moderate	12
	High	13
20s and 30s	Sedentary	10.5
	Moderate	11.5
	High	12.5
40s and 50s	Sedentary	10
	Moderate	11
	High	12
60s and 70s	Sedentary	9.5
	Moderate	10.5
	High	11.5
Over 80	Sedentary	9
	Moderate	10
	High	11

MEN

CARB CHART

Male 5'0" to 5'3" with a desired maintenance weight of 106–136 pounds

Age	Activity	Maximum carb servings/day
Teens–age 20	Sedentary	9
	Moderate	10
	High	11
20s and 30s	Sedentary	8.5
	Moderate	9.5
	High	10.5
40s and 50s	Sedentary	8
	Moderate	9
	High	10

Age	Activity	Maximum carb servings/day
60s and 70s	Sedentary	7.5
	Moderate	8.5
	High	9.5
Over 80	Sedentary	7
	Moderate	8
	High	9

Male 5'4" to 5'7" with a desired maintenance weight of 130–160 pounds

	Activity	Maximum carb servings/day
Teens–age 20	Sedentary	10
	Moderate	11
	High	12
20s and 30s	Sedentary	9.5
	Moderate	10.5
	High	11.5
40s and 50s	Sedentary	9
	Moderate	10
	High	11
60s and 70s	Sedentary	8.5
	Moderate	9.5
	High	10.5
Over 80	Sedentary	8
	Moderate	9
	High	10

Male 5'8" to 5'11" with a desired maintenance weight of 154–185 pounds

	Activity	Maximum carb servings/day
Teens–age 20	Sedentary	11
	Moderate	12
	High	13
20s and 30s	Sedentary	10.5
	Moderate	11.5
	High	12.5

Age	Activity	Maximum carb servings/day
40s and 50s	Sedentary	10
	Moderate	11
	High	12
60s and 70s	Sedentary	9.5
	Moderate	10.5
	High	11.5
Over 80	Sedentary	9
	Moderate	10
	High	11

Male 6'0" to 6'3" with a desired maintenance weight of 178–210 pounds

Age	Activity	Maximum carb servings/day
Teens–age 20	Sedentary	12
	Moderate	13
	High	14
20s and 30s	Sedentary	11.5
	Moderate	12.5
	High	13.5
40s and 50s	Sedentary	11
	Moderate	12
	High	13
60s and 70s	Sedentary	10.5
	Moderate	11.5
	High	12.5
Over 80	Sedentary	10
	Moderate	11
	High	12

Male 6'3" to 6'6" with a desired maintenance weight of 196–235 pounds

Age	Activity	Maximum carb servings/day
Teens–age 20	Sedentary	13
	Moderate	14
	High	15

Age	Activity	Maximum carb servings/day
20s and 30s	Sedentary	12.5
	Moderate	13.5
	High	14.5
40s and 50s	Sedentary	12
	Moderate	13
	High	14
60s and 70s	Sedentary	11.5
	Moderate	12.5
	High	13.5
Over 80	Sedentary	11
	Moderate	12
	High	13

Male over 6'6" with a desired maintenance weight of 226–250 pounds

Teens–age 20	Sedentary	14
	Moderate	15
	High	16
20s and 30s	Sedentary	13.5
	Moderate	14.5
	High	15.5
40s and 50s	Sedentary	13
	Moderate	14
	High	15
60s and 70s	Sedentary	12.5
	Moderate	13.5
	High	14.5
Over 80	Sedentary	12
	Moderate	13
	High	14

Rosa and Jason: One Day in Life of "Their" Step 3

Let's take a look at how a woman who is moving to Step 3 might choose to spread her carb servings throughout the day. Rosa has type 2 diabetes. She is a 45-year-old woman who is 5' 3" and gets moderate physical activity. The chart shows that she can use a maximum amount of 8 carb servings per day.

6:00 AM	Rosa wakes up and checks her blood sugar (she has type 2 diabetes and takes oral medication). She notes her sugar in her log book.
6:30 AM	Breakfast: one carb serving
9:30 AM	Snack: one carb serving (this is needed because the time between her breakfast and lunch exceeds five hours)
1:00 PM	Lunch: two carb servings
4:30 PM	Snack: one carb serving (this is needed because the time between her lunch and dinner exceeds five hours)
7:00 PM	Dinner: two carb servings
9:00 PM	Check blood sugar (Rosa is checking her two-hour post-dinner reading)
11:00 PM	Bedtime: one carb serving

Rosa chose to have eight carb servings, which is her maximum for the day.

Because Step 3 is individualized to height, weight, and activity, the carb requirements for everyone will be different. Jason is 5' 9" inches, 35-year-old man with sedentary physical activity. He was recently diagnosed with type 2 diabetes and is controlling his blood sugar with diet and thirty minutes of walking five times a week. He has a maximum amount of 10.5 carb servings in a day.

6:00 AM	Jason wakes up, checks his blood sugar, and records it in his log book. His reading is 110 mg/dL. He intends to exercise before breakfast, so he eats one 11–20 gram carb serving before he begins his workout
8:30 AM	Breakfast: one carb serving
11:00 AM	Snack of a neutral food (breakfast and lunch fall within five hours of each other)
12:30 PM	Lunch: two carb servings
2:30 PM	Jason checks his blood sugar two hours after lunch
4:00 PM	Snack: one carb serving
6:00 PM	Dinner: three carb servings
11:00 PM	Bedtime: one carb serving

Jason has had nine carb servings, which is within his maximum of 10.5 per day.

These two examples illustrate how Step 3's simple rules were followed:

1. They both consumed their first carb servings within one hour of waking up.
2. Jason ate a carb serving before his early morning exercise.
3. Each meal contains carb servings (no fewer than one serving, no more than four servings).
4. Whenever periods between meals exceed five hours, between-meal snacks contain a carb serving.
5. They had their last carb serving before bed.

As you can see, when you live in Step 3, the program is much more of a lifestyle than a diet. These simple rules become second nature.

FIBER IS YOUR FRIEND

Although a greater variety of carb choices is at your disposal in Step 3, it is always advisable to include higher-fiber choices. The more fiber a food contains, the slower and lower the rise in blood sugar it causes. Higher fiber also helps control cholesterol, speeds food through the GI tract, and is known to help prevent diverticulosis and GI cancers. The chart below will give you an idea of which Step 3 carbohydrates fall into the low-impact zone and those that fall into the less-desirable high-impact zone.

STEP 3 FOOD LISTS

All portions equal one carb serving (11–20 grams of net carbs).

BREADS—LOW IMPACT

Each of the following should have at least 2 grams of fiber.

2 slices of light, thin-sliced whole-grain bread

1 slice of whole-grain bread

1 light whole-grain English muffin

½ whole-grain English muffin

1 light or lower-carb whole-grain pita

½ whole grain pita.

A FOOD SCALE FOR YOUR COUNTERTOP CAN HELP WITH UNLABELED BREAD AND BREAD PRODUCTS

You may want to purchase a simple food scale for bakery bread, homemade bread or rolls, bagels, and chapati. Every ounce of bread is equal to one carb serving (11–20 grams net carb).

DETERMINING HOW MANY CARB SERVINGS ARE CONTAINED IN BREADED FOODS OR FOODS WITH AN "UNKNOWN" SAUCE OR GRAVY

Consider counting breading as one carb serving and sauce of unknown origin (sauce made out of the home and not labeled) as one carb serving. So, a portion of chicken parmesan with marinara sauce would be counted as two carb servings (breading and sauce). Meatballs in sauce would also be counted as two carb servings for the breadcrumbs and sauce.

BREADS—HIGH IMPACT

1 ounce slice of white, whole-wheat, rye, or pumpernickel bread

1 hot dog roll

½ burger bun

½ pita

¾ ounce matzo

1 ounce chapati

1 ounce mini-bagel or mini-muffin

1 fajita shell

1 soft taco shell

2 hard taco shells

1 frozen waffle

2 4-inch pancakes

breading

2 inch cube of corn bread

1 ounce of bakery bread

¾ cup croutons.

CEREALS AND GRAINS—LOW IMPACT

½ cup cooked oatmeal

½ cup cooked barley

½ cup of cooked brown or wild rice

½ cup of cooked whole-grain pasta (al dente)

½ cup cooked bulgur

½ cup cooked quinoa.

CEREALS AND GRAINS—HIGH IMPACT

½ cup cooked cream of wheat

½ cup cooked farina

½ cup cooked grits

⅓ cup cooked white rice

½ cup basmati rice

⅓ cup cooked white pasta

½ cup of pasta salad

½ cup of macaroni and cheese

½ cup casserole dish made with pasta.

CRACKERS AND STARCHY SNACKS—LOW IMPACT

Be sure to check labels to ensure you are consuming 11–20 grams of net carbs, no trans fats, and at least 2 grams of fiber.

A serving of crackers with the appropriate carbs and fiber

3 cups popcorn (light or air-popped without partially hydrogenated oils)

Whole-grain pretzels

Corn tortilla chips.

CRACKERS AND STARCHY SNACKS—HIGH IMPACT

Snacks are high impact, even if you eat the appropriate serving amount, if they do not have adequate fiber.

A serving of crackers containing 11–20 grams carb.

Chips

Pretzels

1 ½ oblong graham crackers (3 squares)

4 slices of melba toast

2 large rice cakes

8 small rice cakes

6 saltines

½ cup chow mein noodles

3 sandwich crackers with cheese or peanut butter filling.

STARCHY VEGETABLES/LEGUMES—LOW IMPACT

½ cup of corn

½ ear of fresh corn

½ cup of peas

½ cup of legumes, such as kidney beans, lentils, lima beans, chickpeas, white beans, black beans, and white kidney beans

⅓ cup of hummus

½ sweet potato or yam

½ cup of mashed sweet potato or yam

1 ½ cup of cooked carrots

1 cup of beets.

STARCHY VEGETABLES/LEGUMES—HIGH IMPACT

½ cup mashed potatoes

½ baked white potato

½ (3 ounces) of boiled potato

½ small order of French fries

1/3 cup baked beans

½ cup potato salad

½ cup mashed plantain

1 cup winter squash

1 cup canned pumpkin.

SOUPS—LOW IMPACT

1 cup of tomato soup (water-based)

½ cup lentil soup

½ cup split pea soup.

1 cup of meat chili with beans.

SOUPS—HIGH IMPACT

1 cup of broth-based soup with noodles, potatoes, rice, and barley

1 cup of cream soup

½ cup of pasta e fagioli

1 cup of greens and beans

½ cup of minestrone soup

PROTEIN AND CEREAL BARS—LOW IMPACT

To be low impact, a protein bar must contain 11–20 grams of net carbs and have 2 grams or more of fiber.

PROTEIN AND CEREAL BARS—HIGH IMPACT

A high-impact protein bar is any that contains 11–20 grams of net carbs and less than 2 grams of fiber.

FRUIT—LOW IMPACT

All portions represent 11–20 grams of net carbs. Fruit choices should be average in size.

1 apple or 4 apple rings

1 pear

1 peach

2 plums

1 nectarine

12 cherries

½ cup of natural applesauce

½ grapefruit (not allowed with Lipitor)

1 cup of whole strawberries (approximately 6–8 berries)

¾ cup of blackberries

¾ cup of blueberries

1 cup of raspberries

2 clementine oranges or 2 small tangerines

8 dried apricot halves or 4 apricots

12 grapes

1 orange

¾ cup of pineapple cubes

½ banana

1 cup melon (canteloupe, honeydew, watermelon).

FRUIT—HIGH IMPACT

3 dates

2 figs

1 kiwi

¾ cup mandarin oranges

½ small or ½ cup mango

1 cup papaya cubes or ½ papaya

2 prunes

2 tablespoons of raisins

MILK AND OTHER DAIRY—LOW IMPACT

All portions represent 11–20 grams carbs.

1 cup (8 fluid ounces) of fat-free, 1, or 2 percent milk

Plain yogurt

Fruit-flavored yogurt sweetened with sucralose

½ cup of sugar-free/fat-free pudding

No-sugar-added ice cream.

MILK AND OTHER DAIRY—HIGH IMPACT

½ cup ice cream (light, low-fat, regular)

½ cup frozen yogurt (light or regular).

OCCASIONAL TREATS

Treats and sweets are high-impact carbs that are often high in fat and have little nutritional benefit. Still, they can be a tasty treat from time to time. Below are typical serving sizes with the carb servings listed beside them. Try not to have two treats in one day because they have a high glycemic index and shoot your blood sugar up very quickly. A good rule of thumb is a max of two treats per week.

Brownie, 4 inch square, unfrosted: 2 carb servings
Brownie, 4 inch square, frosted: 4 carb servings
Cake, 4 inch square, unfrosted: 2 carb servings
Cake, 4 inch square, frosted: 4 carb servings
2 sandwich-type cookies with filling in the middle: 1 carb serving
2 cookies, average size, homemade, such as chocolate chip: 1 carb
    serving
Frosted cupcake (small): 2 carb servings
Plain cake doughnut: 2 carb servings
Glazed-type doughnut: 2 carb servings
Fruit pie with 2 crusts (⅛ pie): 3 carb servings
⅛ single-crusted fruit pie: 2 carb servings
⅛ pumpkin or custard pie: 2 carb servings
⅛ large pizza: 3 carb servings
⅛ large pizza, thick outer edge of crust removed: 2 carb servings
Bagel: 4 carb servings
½ bagel: 2 carb servings
"Hollowed bagel" with insides scooped out: 2 carb servings
Hard roll, kaiser roll, 6" inch sub roll: 3 carb servings
"Hollowed" hard roll, kaiser roll, sub roll: 2 carb servings
Wrap: 3 carb servings
1 cup casserole dishes, such as lasagna, macaroni and cheese, or
    tuna casserole: 2 carb servings

Small fries: 2 carb servings

Medium fries: 3 carb servings

Large fries: 4 carb servings

Breaded fish sandwich on a bun: 3 carb servings

Breaded chicken on a bun: 3 carb servings

Bun for large burgers or fast food sandwiches: 3 carb servings

Chicken nuggets, 6 pack: 1 carb serving

Sushi, 6 pieces: 1 carb serving

Chinese food, such as beef and broccoli or shrimp and veggies
    with sauce (no rice or noodles), 1 cup: 1 carb serving

Chinese rice, white or fried, 1 cup: 3 carb servings

Chinese lo mein noodles, 1 cup: 2 carb servings

2 wontons: 1 carb serving

Sauce or breading on any food: 1 carb serving

SAMPLE MENUS FOR STEP 3

BREAKFAST: 2 CARB SERVING

Egg white omelet with baby spinach, tomatoes, and feta cheese

1 light multigrain English muffin (1 carb serving)

Whipped butter

1 cup cubed honeydew (1 carb serving)

Coffee with light creamer.

2 whole-grain waffles (2 carb servings)

Light whipped cream

Zero-carb syrup

Coffee with creamer.

Scrambled eggs mixed with cubed baked ham

1 multigrain bagel thin (1 carb serving)

(continued)

Whipped butter

½ grapefruit (1 carb serving)

Green tea with stevia.

¾ cup Greek yogurt (1 carb serving)

6 sliced strawberries (1 carb serving)

Flavored water.

¾ cup of Cheerios (1 carb serving)

1 cup 1 percent milk (1 carb serving)

Herbal tea with lemon.

½ cup cooked oatmeal (1 carb serving)

Unsweetened almond or soy milk

½ banana (1 carb serving).

1 slice multigrain toast (1 carb serving)

Whipped butter

Dip of ricotta cheese

1 kiwi, sliced (1 carb serving).

LUNCH: 2 CARB SERVINGS

2 slices of light whole-wheat bread (1 carb serving)

Oven-baked roast beef

Sliced low-fat cheese

Romaine lettuce and tomato slices

Spicy mustard

1 pear (1 carb serving)

Diet drink.

½ cup pea soup (1 carb serving)
Crackers (amount that contains 11–20 grams net carb = 1 carb
    serving)
Cobb salad with light ranch dressing
Sparkling water.

1 cup chicken noodle soup (1 carb serving)
Tuna salad on 2 slices light multigrain toast (1 carb serving)
Sugar-free iced tea with lemon wedge.

Fajitas ordered in a restaurant (chicken/beef/shrimp, shredded
    cheese, lettuce, tomato, pico de gallo, guacamole, onions, and
    peppers
2 6-inch fajita wraps (2 carb servings)
Diet drink.

1 slice pizza (take back crust off) (2 carb servings) with cheese and
    veggies
Antipasta salad: romaine lettuce, roasted peppers, artichoke hearts,
    olives, peperoncini, cherry tomatoes, and balsamic vinaigrette
Sugar-free drink.

Chef's salad with turkey, roast beef, and cheese
Light Caesar dressing
2 ounce dinner roll (2 carb servings)
Whipped butter
Lemon water.

Burger bun (2 carb servings)
Grilled sirloin burger
Cheesy chips (see page 158)
Grilled mushrooms
Iced green tea with lemon.

Eggplant parmesan (2 carb servings for breading and sauce)
Caesar salad without croutons
Water.

Light yogurt (1 carb serving)
2 chocolate chip cookies with 11–20 grams carb (1 carb serving)
Decaf iced coffee with creamer.

DINNER: 3 CARB SERVINGS

Breaded chicken cutlets (1 carb serving for breading)
1 cup mashed potatoes (2 carb servings)
Garden green beans
Sparkling water with lime.

5 ounces red wine
Sirloin tips with gravy (1 carb serving for gravy)
1 cup whole-grain lightly buttered noodles (2 carb servings)
Green beans almondine
Iced coffee with creamer and stevia.

Tuna salad–stuffed tomato
2 ounce slice of multigrain bakery bread (2 carb servings)
6 strawberries with whipped cream (1 carb serving)
Iced ginger tea.

White wine
Grilled chicken
Baked potato (2 carb servings)
Whipped butter, light sour cream, and chives
Sautéed brussels sprouts
2 oatmeal cookies (1 carb serving)
Herbal tea and lemon.

Roast pork loin
½ cup natural applesauce (1 carb serving)
½ cup mashed potatoes (1 carb serving)
½ cup corn (1 carb serving)
Diet drink.

Baked ham
Roasted sweet potato (2 carb servings)
Steamed cauliflower
½ cup light chocolate ice cream (1 carb serving)
Sugar-free beverage.

1 cup tomato soup (1 carb serving)
1 cup macaroni and cheese (2 carb servings)
Greek salad with feta cheese and olives
Diet drink.

"Breakfast for Dinner"
1 cup fruit salad (1 carb serving)
Poached egg and turkey sausage on a multigrain light English
    muffin (1 carb serving)
1 cup 1 percent milk (1 carb serving).

How to Manage Slip-ups on Step 3

As you learned in Step 2, it is possible to have a dietary indiscretion as long as you keep track of the number of mistakes in a week and then reset effectively.

Step 3 gives you so much freedom, variety, and flexibility that it is very likely that you will not have many slip-ups. Step 3 is not a weight-loss phase . . . it is a weight- and health-maintenance phase. You have

Sick Day Guidelines for Diabetes

During illness, the body releases hormones to help fight the infection. A side effect of these hormones is a dramatic rise in blood sugar. Some people report that their blood sugar begins to rise 1–2 days before they experience the first symptoms of an illness. Continue to take diabetes oral medications or insulin even if you cannot eat as your blood sugar rises from the illness.

If you have a drop in blood sugar after vomiting or diarrhea, call your MD as medications may be suspended until you can keep food down. Treat hypoglycemia as described on pages (294–295). It is more likely that your blood sugar will be elevated during illness. It is a good idea to talk to your doctor about sick day instructions before you are sick!

When Ill, It Is Recommended That You:
1. Test and record your blood sugar at least every 4 hours.
2. Check and record your body temperature every 4 hours.
3. Drink, drink, drink! You need at least 4 ounces of decaf, carb-free fluid every hour if you don't have a fever and at least 8 ounces/hour if you have a fever (temperature over 99.5 degrees)

   Examples: water, sugar-free sports drinks (contain electrolytes), decaf or herbal tea, broth, sugar-free jello, sugar-free ice pops, carb-free/caffeine-free drinks. It is very important for people with diabetes to stay hydrated when they are ill as dehydration can cause serious consequences.
4. Eat appropriately for the Step of the program you are on. It may be better to hit your carb targets with liquids or easy to swallow foods if you are experiencing nausea or vomiting.
5. Focus on carb-free liquids only if your blood sugar is over 250. There is no need to hit carb targets as your blood sugar is already elevated.
6. Call your doctor if vomiting or diarrhea lasts over 24 hours, if you have a high fever (over 101.5 degrees) for over 24 hours, or if you have extreme fatigue, shortness of breath, dizziness, or pain.
7. Do a urine test for ketones every 4 hours if your blood sugar is over 250 and you are taking insulin. Urine ketostix can be purchased non-prescription at your pharmacy. Consult with your doctor if blood sugar exceeds 300 and/or if urine ketones exceed 2+ (moderate).

What To Do About Diabetes Medication If You Are Sick?
Never skip your diabetes medication when you are sick. You may actually need more medication or even insulin to normalize high blood sugars caused by illness.

(continues)

(continued)

Metformin:

1. Don't take metformin until you can keep food and liquids down.
2. If you have symptoms of lactic acidosis: muscle weakness, sleepiness, slow heart rate, muscle pain, shortness of breath, stomach pain, fainting . . . report to your M.D. immediately.
3. If you are having surgery or a dye injected study: check with your M.D. as you might need to stop taking metformin before the procedure.

Oral Medication for Diabetes During Illness:

1. Take your medications as directed.
2. If you think you vomited the pills, don't take more medication and report this to your doctor.
3. Sometimes your MD will temporarily prescribe insulin if blood sugar is significantly elevated from illness.

Insulin Usage During Illness

1. The full dose of daily insulin is usually required.
2. If your blood sugar is **high**, you may need to take frequent doses of rapid-acting insulin to normalize the readings.
3. If your blood sugar is **too low**, your physician may advise you to stop taking rapid acting insulin until your blood sugar normalizes and you can keep fluids down.
4. If you have questions or are not sure about the right thing to do, call your doctor for instructions.

the choice to eat anywhere in the carb range. However, just like in Step 2, if you find that you have more than two dietary slip-ups in a week on Step 3, return to Step 1 for ten days, followed by ten days in Step 2, and then resume Step 3. Always follow a detox in Step 1 by an equal or greater amount of time in Step 2 before returning to Step 3.

For example, if after vacation, holidays, or a long weekend in which you were off of your Step 3 maintenance plan more than twice, you should return to ten days of Step 1 and ten days of Step 2. During high-stress times, including emotional stress, before or after surgery, and illness or pain that lasts more than three days, it is always safest to go back to Step 1. High levels of stress, both emotional and physical, may upset your insulin balance. Illness and pain can hike blood sugar numbers and stress the pancreas. When your health or stress issue is resolved, begin ten days of Step 1, followed by an equal amount of time in Step 2 before going back to Step 3.

FREQUENTLY ASKED QUESTIONS FOR STEP 3

I understand that I have greater freedom in Step 3; there will be a larger carb range and more variety. What can I do to ensure that my weight does, indeed, maintain?

As long as you stay within the recommended amount of carb servings to maintain your desired weight for height and activity, you will not overstimulate the pancreas, turn on insulin, send blood sugar rocketing, or gain weight from carbs. Your carbs are set at your maintenance weight. Spread them out according to the rules of Step 3 and live your life.

In addition to paying attention to your carb intake, you should always select reasonable portions of low–fat healthy proteins and heart-healthy fats, limit the overuse of salt, drink adequate fluids, and exercise regularly.

I'm perfectly happy with the amount of carbohydrates I have in Step 2. My blood sugar is perfect, and my physician has eliminated my medication for diabetes, cholesterol, and blood pressure. What will happen if I continue with the carb allotment for Step 2? Must I increase my carbs to my maintenance amount?

The rules of Step 3 show you the range of carbs that would be acceptable; The low end is one carb serving per meal or necessary snack, and the high end is dependent on your individual needs. You may absolutely take the lower end of the range of carbohydrates for your body (see the chart on page 213–218) but realize that going to the maximum will not trigger weight gain. You should strive to achieve the middle ground of carb grams in your target range for meals and snacks.

If you are comfortable living with 11–20 grams of carbs at meals and snacks that require a carb counter, be liberal with your lean protein and heart-healthy fat intake to maintain your weight. Step 2 is, after all, a weight-loss phase.

I would recommend that you consider the mind-set of Step 3 for the long term. You can certainly choose to eat at the lower end of your range, but you may also find that you would occasionally enjoy a day or two per week at the higher end of your range.

I spent eight weeks on Step 1, twenty-four weeks in Step 2, and have maintained my desired weight for more than a year on Step 3. My blood sugar readings are always in the normal range, and I have been able to eliminate all diabetes medications. I've cured my type 2 diabetes, right? Is it safe to go back to eating like I used to, before I began the Diabetes Miracle?

Despite what you might have read, you can't cure type 2 diabetes, just as you can't cure your genetic makeup. If you return to your pre-program way of life, the metabolic mayhem will restart, and you will find yourself gaining weight, with rising blood sugar and declining energy levels. Step 3 is a way of life designed for the health and well-being of anyone with Met B, prediabetes, or diabetes. It gives you great freedom in carb amount and variety. Though you won't cure your diabetes, you will be in control of your diabetes.

Step 3 has been great. I'm at my desired weight, and my blood sugar is under control. But lately I've noticed my clothes are feeling tight, and my fasting blood sugar has been getting higher. What can I do to correct this problem?

When you find that undesired changes are happening, it's time to take a close look at how you are following the program. An easy way to assess how well you are adhering to Step 3 is to keep a food log detailing the foods you eat and the times you eat them. Be sure to include approximate portion sizes and the carb grams in your foods. Write down your fluid intake, vitamins and minerals, and exercise. Don't forget to note how you are feeling—if you are under high stress, are ill, or have significant pain.

After the third complete day, carefully review your log and see how well it matches up to the rules for Step 3:

- Am I eating the appropriate amount of carbohydrate within one hour of waking up?
- Am I taking a night snack with the appropriate amount of carb grams at bedtime?
- Do I take an appropriate carb snack if I awaken in the middle of the night?
- Am I eating the right amount of carbs before early morning exercise?
- If the time between my meals exceeds five hours, do I take the correct amount of carbs at my between-meals snack?
- Am I eating carbohydrates at each meal and appropriate snack?
- Am I exercising a minimum of thirty minutes, five times/week? Is it time to change up my exercise routine?
- Am I drinking adequate water/decaf liquid?

If you have been following the rules to a "T," there may be something else going on. Ask yourself:

- Am I going through a period of high stress?
- Am I ill, recovering from surgery or an illness, or temporarily using a steroid-based medication such as prednisone?
- Am I in significant pain?

If you answered "no" to the above, your life is fairly stable, and nothing is causing you pain, uncontrolled Met B is most likely not the cause of your recent increase in weight. Your weight gain may be because of excess consumption of protein and fat. Take a closer look at your portion sizes, and perhaps decrease your intake of added fat, such as butter, cream cheese, salad dressing, cream, oil, fatty meats, deli meats, high-fat cheeses, and poultry skin.

Perhaps you misread a label for carb grams. Some manufacturers purposely indicate lower-than-reality carb grams on the front of their packaging, but a look at the nutrition facts shows these foods really contain far more carb grams. Eating these foods could cause weight gain and blood sugar increase.

If you are adhering to the lifestyle plan, are not experiencing stress or illness, and are not overeating neutral foods, ask your physician to consider checking your thyroid panel, cortisol level, and serum insulin. It is rare, but another metabolic issue may be at play.

I know that both emotional and physical stress causes stress hormones to increase, which raises my blood sugar, which causes my diabetes and weight to go out of control. I understand that Step 1 is the safest place to be when under stress. But my stress is going to be long-term. I just got divorced and am a single parent to three teenagers. I also have chronic back pain from a car accident three years ago. What are my options to get control of my diabetes and weight despite my high-stress life?

You certainly do have your share of stress, and you are correct in assessing that this is going to be a long-term stressful time (three teenagers!).

Your first option is to live in Step 1, and because you are doing it for a longer period of time, give yourself one five-hour block "off" per week. This will make Step 1 more livable.

The second is to do a four-week rehab/detox in Step 1 and before you move to Steps 2 or 3, ask your doctor about possibly prescribing the diabetes medication metformin. Metformin works to decrease the liver's release of blood sugar when you exceed five hours without a carb, during the night while you are asleep, and during times of stress.

In Step 1, your liver was emptied of blood sugar stores. In Steps 2 and 3, your liver is filled with glycogen and will react to gaps between meals, sleep time, and stress with an overflow of glycogen. Metformin helps to decrease the amount of the glycogen release, which in turn helps to decrease insulin resistance.

I am pleased that I can occasionally have some "empty-calorie" carb treats, such as cookies, candy, ice cream, and marshmallows, while on Step 3. If I make sure they fit into my allotted net carb amount, how often can I choose these sweet treats?

Not only does the amount of carbohydrates impact insulin release, but the type of carb also has an effect. If you have a small frozen gelato (45 grams of carbohydrate, thus a three carb serving) at the end of a carb-free dinner of grilled chicken, sautéed veggies, and garden salad, it will make blood sugar spike hard and fast. (Note that if your three carb servings came from ½ cup chickpeas added to your salad and an ear of corn, your blood sugar rise would be slower and smoother.)

Immediately after eating dessert, your pancreas was triggered by the immediate request for a lot of insulin. But, if that same 45 grams of carbs came from lower-glycemic carb grams, you blood sugar would rise to a reasonable height at an easy pace, keeping the pancreas relaxed.

Try to limit the use of empty-calorie carbs to no more than twice a week, and don't eat more than one on the same day. By using these foods as occasional treats, you will treat your body well and maintain your desired health goals.

> *My husband and I both have type 2 diabetes. We have had a great time following Steps 1 and 2 together. Our blood sugar is terrific, we feel great, our lab work has improved, and we are both at our desired weight. Amazingly, we were able to follow the same program, although he is 58 years of age, is 5 feet 11 inches tall, and now weighs 178 pounds. I am 48 years old, am 5 feet 5 inches tall, and now weigh 148 pounds. We are both happy with our body size and want to begin Step 3. Is there a Step 3 that we can do together? We don't want to be on different plans for life!*

People are always surprised that no matter the gender, starting weight, age, or medication package, everyone does Step 1 for eight weeks (some people stay longer). At the end of the eighth week, everyone does Step 2 for at least eight weeks or until reaching the desired size and being on as little medication as possible.

When it comes to Step 3, your lifetime program, you will always be eating a different amount of carb grams than your husband. You will have less carb servings a day because you are different in all the ways you point out.

Because you both desire to maintain your different weights given your different genders, heights, and ages, the amount of carbohydrates in your target ranges has to be different. I suggest focusing on the similarities: Are you on the same lifestyle program? Yes. Will you both follow the same rules? Yes. Are you both in Step 3 of the Diabetes Miracle? Yes. Will you eat the same foods? Yes, if you want to. The only difference will be that your husband's carb range to maintain his weight will be higher than yours.

I have had tremendous success on the Diabetes Miracle. My A1C dropped from 8.0 to 6.5. My LDL decreased from 156 to 90. My blood pressure is now normal. My vitamin D level rose from 28 to 46. My issue is that my physician refuses to address the fact that I'm still taking medication for blood sugar, cholesterol, and blood pressure despite these improved readings. She told me that the reason my readings are improved is because of my medications. What can I do to convince her otherwise?

Never eliminate prescribed medications without physician approval. Some medications need to be gradually decreased, not quickly eliminated, and others might be in place for reasons other than the obvious (for example, some blood pressure medications, called ACE inhibitors, have the ability to take pressure off the kidneys, so some physicians prescribe them preventatively).

You need to have a short talk with your doctor and ask her if she would consider decreasing or eliminating a medication as long as you continue on the Diabetes Miracle and return for follow-up at an appointed time to assess how you are faring on diet and exercise without the medication. She may work on one medication at a time. In time, your cholesterol, blood pressure, blood sugar, and vitamin D may be maintained on diet and exercise alone . . . or you may require a smaller dose of your medications.

You must realize that until now, physicians were not accustomed to seeing patients with type 2 diabetes or prediabetes making such amazing changes in their bodies and medication requirements. You will be able to objectively show her proof with future lab tests/pressure readings/blood glucose self-monitoring, weights, and body measurements.

Step 3 will soon become a way of life. Even though you will live on Step 3, you will always have all three steps of the Diabetes Miracle to work with throughout life. You will use Step 1 whenever you need to reset the pancreas/liver combination. Step 2 will always bridge Steps 1 and 3 as it retrains the pancreas to handle carbohydrates. And Step 3 will enable you to live the life you desire and deserve with flexibility and ease.

Part Three

THE DIABETES MIRACLE LIFESTYLE

EXERCISE: MAKING THE TIME TO GET FIT

After thirty years of working with people on their diet and lifestyle programs, I've come to realize that the word *exercise* conjures up very different reactions. There are the people who are devoted exercisers, who would not dream of forgoing a gym day. By contrast, the majority of people I've counseled understand the need to become physically active, but tend to have difficulty committing to an active lifestyle. When I first meet patients, more than 75 percent get no regular exercise.

The number one reason people list for not being more active is lack of time. Many view exercise as work—just one more thing that must be scheduled into a busy day, which will take up a block of valuable time in an already cramped schedule. These people often find fitting in exercise to be more difficult than the diet aspect of their program.

Young and middle-aged people commute to school or work, have very busy days, and often bring home projects to be completed in the evening. Add children or other family members to this mix, and it becomes easy to see why exercise might slip through the cracks.

Older people may find themselves dealing with aches and pains, preexisting medical conditions, fatigue, and fear of falling. Sometimes they don't know how to safely exercise.

A DIFFERENT TAKE ON PHYSICAL ACTIVITY

We all have our reasons for not exercising, but just as a person needs to sleep and eat, he needs to be physically active to maintain a healthy body and mind. Good health is fueled with nourishing food, adequate sleep, and physical activity.

Although many people view exercise as just one more thing to do, almost no one views eating dinner or climbing into bed at night as one more time-consuming task. Somehow, although it is as essential as food or rest, exercise has become optional.

In the past, people did not have to plan exercise. Their everyday lives were physically active because activity was a way of life. Most chores were done manually, clothes were washed in ringer washers and hung outside to dry, jobs revolved around physical labor, people walked to and from school or work, children played outdoors from morning until nightfall, housework could take up an entire day, and yard work could consume an entire weekend.

Today's lifestyle is markedly different from the lifestyles of our parents and grandparents. Many jobs involve sitting down at a computer for long stretches of time, and we commute to work by driving our cars door to door or by taking public transportation. We use remote controls rather than get up to change the channel on the television and sit in front of the TV or computer every evening while our children play passively indoors with video and computer games or communicate on their cell phones. Appliances do much of our physical work. Many hire others to do yard work, or we use a ride-on mower, and snow is removed with snowblowers or plows. As a result, if we don't take the time and make an effort to exercise, there can be entire weeks, months, or years in which we get no significant physical activity.

The human body was never meant to be physically inactive. Your muscles are meant to spend their glycogen stores and get refilled with blood sugar on a daily basis. The act of exercise allows muscle tissue to break down a bit and rebuild/rejuvenate, thus keeping the muscle metabolically active and toned. Exercise is necessary to keep the heart muscle healthy, to keep the lungs breathing to capacity, and to help food move through the GI tract. Without exercise, our blood sugar and insulin levels rise, blood pressure elevates, and our metabolic rate slows. Without exercise, we have no immediate outlet for the anxiety and stress caused by the times in which we live—the fight-or-flight response offers a lot of fight (stress hormones) without much flight (activity).

EIGHT BENEFITS OF EXERCISE FOR PEOPLE WITH DIABETES

Everyone knows that physical activity and exercise are important to maintain a healthy body and mind. But if you have Met B, prediabetes, or type 2 diabetes, you stand to benefit even more from exercise than the average person. Exercise can benefit you in the following ways.

1. **Reduce weight:** If you have Met B, losing as little as 7 percent of your body weight results in substantial reductions in blood pressure, glucose, triglycerides, and total cholesterol—all factors that can lead to heart disease. A 180-pound woman who loses 12 pounds makes a huge difference in her present and future health and well-being.
2. **Decreases insulin resistance:** The act of exercise moves sugar from the bloodstream directly into muscle cells, leaving less sugar in the blood to trigger insulin release. As fat cells decrease in size, insulin fits receptors better. In this way, exercise helps decrease our insulin resistance.
3. **Immediate and time-released decreases in blood sugar:** Exercise immediately decreases blood sugar and stimulates cells to uptake blood sugar for hours after the exercise is complete.
4. **Reduces blood pressure:** Regular exercise strengthens the heart, blood vessels, and cardiovascular system and promotes fat-burning

and weight loss, all of which help lower blood pressure. Exercise helps keep your arteries flexible, which helps prevent heart disease and heart attacks.

5. **Reduces stress, relieves anxiety, and reduces depression:** The act of exercise blunts the negative effects of stress hormones (decreases stress hormones' ability to raise blood sugar) and helps increase such feel-good hormones as serotonin.

6. **Enhances self-esteem:** A body that is in shape looks and feels younger and sexier, positively affecting self-esteem and body image.

7. **Improves lung capacity:** Aerobic exercise helps the relationship between the heart, blood vessels, and lungs and improves your respiratory capacity.

8. **Boosts immunity:** A body in good physical condition has an enhanced ability to fight infections through improved circulation and normalized blood sugar levels.

MEDICAL CLEARANCE

Get medical clearance before beginning an exercise program if you are experiencing:

- Unusually high blood sugar readings (a significant increase above your normal readings)
- Blood sugar readings close to or more than 300 mg/dL
- Recurring bouts of hypoglycemia
- Chest pain
- Irregular, rapid, or fluttery heart beat
- Shortness of breath
- Significant, ongoing weight loss that hasn't been diagnosed
- Fever
- Deep vein thrombosis (DVT)
- A hernia that is causing symptoms
- Foot or ankle sores that won't heal
- Persistent pain after you have had a fall
- Certain eye conditions, such as bleeding in the retina or detached retina.

Exercising Within the Flow of Your Normal Day: Small Steps to a Big Goal

I'd like to suggest thinking of physical activity as a daily necessity—something your body requires, just at it requires air and food and rest. If you do not currently exercise, this would be a good time to spend a few moments looking at your daily routine to find niches of time where exercise can be inserted into the flow of your day.

I'm sure you've heard that walking is one of the best forms of exercise. It is inexpensive (all you need is a good pair of walking shoes), does not take up space in your home, requires no membership to the gym, and can be done at your convenience.

STEP BY STEP

Typically, when people think of starting a walking program, they try to find a large block of time over and above their normal daily activities to fit the walk in. Because some people have busy schedules with work, home, kids/families, they sometimes postpone starting a walking program thinking that they can't possibly make it happen.

One cool way to increase activity involves a simple gadget that can be purchased in the sporting goods department of any chain store or even in many supermarkets: a pedometer. When you wear a pedometer, it keeps track of exactly how many steps you take. (There are pedometer apps for some cell phones.)

Instead of adding a thirty-minute walk to your day first thing in the morning or at the end of the day, you can add steps into your day. Here's how:

First, determine your baseline. Wear the pedometer for seven days consecutively (weekdays and weekend included). Attach it to your waistband at the start of your day and remove it when you are changing for bed at night. At the end of each day, keep track of the number of steps you took, and reset the pedometer for the next day. At the end of seven days, determine an average of the steps.

For example:

Day 1 = 2,500 steps
Day 2 = 4,000 steps
Day 3 = 3,600 steps
Day 4 = 2,200 steps
Day 5 = 6,000 steps
Day 6 = 4,150 steps
Day 7 = 2,300 steps
Total steps = 24,750

Divided by seven days, and that's an average of 3,535 steps/day in the course of a normal day's activities.

How far did you walk? Well, 2,000 pedometer steps equals approximately one mile, so in the course of the week, you walked close to two miles without expending any extra effort or carving out any extra time. All you need to do is build on those small steps.

For the next week, walk 500 more steps each day. Every 500 steps you take adds an extra one-quarter mile to your day. So, every day for seven days, add 500 steps to your daily total, making sure you exceed 4,000 steps each day.

This slow but steady approach of adding 500 steps a day means you will be adding 1.7 miles to your weekly walking. By systematically building on the number of steps you take each day, you will help to build a healthier body.

Think of it this way: Week 1 = goal of more than 4,000 steps a day adds another 1.7 miles to your week = 1.7 miles over your norm.

Week 2 = goal of more than 4,500 steps a day adds another 1.7 miles = 3.4 miles over your norm.

Week 3 = goal of more than 5,000 steps a day adds another 1.7 miles = 5.1 miles over your norm.

Week 4 = goal of more than 5,500 steps a day adds another 1.7 miles = 6.8 miles over your norm. This step-by-step approach will have you walking seven extra miles a week!

Feel free to get creative about adding extra steps into your day instead of stressing about having to add something at the end of the day. I guarantee that you will find yourself adding some of the following steps to up the pedometer reading.

- Take a walk with your spouse, child, coworker, or friend
- Walk the dog . . . really walk the dog!
- Use the stairs instead of the elevator
- Park farther away from the store or your office
- Get up to change the channel
- Get up to get a glass of water, the pepper shaker, or a cup of tea instead of asking a family member to do it for you
- Window shop in a mall (a great one to do in inclement weather)
- Plan a walking meeting
- Walk over to visit a neighbor
- Get outside to walk around the garden or do a little weeding
- Walk to confer with a coworker rather than send an email
- Get up during work and actually go to the restroom
- Get up during work to get water, to make copies, to stretch your legs, and to collect your thoughts.

The pedometer approach is a wonderful way to start an exercise program based on your actual lifestyle. One person may begin walking only 1,200 steps a day, whereas another person may initially walk 6,000 steps a day. This method enables you to begin at an individual starting point and finish when you are hitting the number of miles per week you want to add into your life.

After a period of time, it will be important to change up your activity by walking faster, farther, on different surfaces, or on different inclines. (See page 333 for a chart to keep track of steps.)

OTHER WAYS TO ADD ACTIVITY INTO YOUR NORMAL DAY

For those who don't wish to take the pedometer approach, there are other ways to incorporate increased activity into your normal day. See if any of the following appeals to you:

- Walk around your office during conference calls or around your house when you are on the phone
- Use light weights during phone or conference calls
- Purchase a small cycling machine that fits under the desk (pedal while you work)
- Start a Walking Club at lunchtime
- Walk around the office building or parking lot before you begin work and before you leave for the day
- Use television commercials to your benefit. A one-hour television program has about fifteen minutes of commercials. Every time commercials interrupt your program, engage in an activity: lift light weights, stretch, march in place, or do squats or lunges. By working out during commercials, after two hours of programming, you will have accomplished one-half hour of activity. This is a much better use of commercial time than zoning out or grabbing a snack.

By incorporating some of these easy ideas, you complete your activity within your normal daily routine and do not have to make time for working out after work or in the evening.

ADDING EXERCISE TO YOUR DAY

Some people prefer to concentrate on their work during their workday and carve out designated time devoted to their exercise regimen before work or at the end of the day. Outdoor walking, playing basketball, tennis, rollerblading, bicycling, gardening, running, jogging, or going to the gym are all forms of exercise that can be enjoyed outside of your work environment. They can provide a much-needed break from the day and add a daily source of fun and enjoyment.

Whether you incorporate the activity into your day, or set aside a block of time, the number one form of exercise chosen by adults is walking. Let's talk about starting a walking program, especially if you haven't done concerted walking in awhile.

THREE WEEKS TO A HABIT

It's been said that it takes a person three weeks for a new activity to become a habit. Consider the first three weeks of exercise as a way for exercise to become a regular part of your life, and take this time to start slowly and gradually work up to a moderate pace and distance. Put on your walking shoes or sneakers and walk out the door. If you are new to walking, start with walking for ten minutes in one direction, then turn around and walk back for ten minutes. That's all there is to it . . . you've just begun a walking program.

If this amount of time was easy for you, add five minutes to your walks on a weekly basis. A twenty-minute walk on week one becomes a twenty-five–minute walk for week two and a thirty-minute walk for week three.

Start your walk at a slower pace (five minutes to warm up). Then, pick up your pace in the middle (twenty minutes of moderate walking), and slow down to cool down (five minutes) toward the end. Make sure to gently stretch after your walk when your muscles are warmed up.

THE BENEFITS OF WALKING

If your goal is to use walking to lower blood sugar, improve blood pressure, and decrease stress, consider walking a minimum of thirty minutes a day, five days a week, at a "talking" pace (the pace at which you can still carry on a conversation without becoming short of breath).

If your goal is to achieve the above plus to improve your cardiovascular fitness, you should walk five days a week, a minimum of forty minutes at a brisk pace—breathing harder but not gasping for air. As always, warm up at the beginning and slow down at the end (for five minutes each).

If your goal is all of the above plus weight loss, you should walk a minimum of five days a week for forty-five to sixty minutes at a brisk pace, including warm-up and cool-down mode.

Once you are comfortable reaching your goal time and days a week, you may want to either ramp up your speed, add five minutes to the walk, carry light hand weights, or change your route to include more inclines. The body gets accustomed to the "same ol', same ol'," so make sure to occasionally vary your walking routine by changing the time spent or the intensity of your walk.

HOW TO RAMP UP YOUR WALK
WITHOUT INCREASING THE TIME FACTOR

If you want to change up your walk but do not want to add more time, consider the following ways to add some zip to your thirty-minute allotment for exercise:

- Pick up your pace: Walk a little faster. Some people eventually work up to the speed of racewalking.
- Pump it up: When you pump your arms during your walk, you get more cardiovascular benefit and burn more calories.
- Head for the hills: Add some hills to your daily thirty-minute walk, or increase the incline on your treadmill.

- Add some weight: Carrying light hand weights adds resistance and intensity to your walk.
- Change the surface: Consider occasionally changing the surface that you walk on. Walking on a track, on a sidewalk, in sand, through water, or on gravel or a dirt surface actually changes up your half-hour walk while giving you a change of scenery.

GETTING THE RIGHT AMOUNT OF CARDIO FITNESS FROM YOUR WORKOUT

According to the American Heart Association (AHA), it's important to pace yourself during exercise. Overdoing your program can cause you to tire quickly or become injured from doing too much, too soon. Alternatively, not exerting yourself enough will not give you the desired heart-healthy benefits. There are two primary methods of assessing if the level at which you are walking is correct for you.

The Talk Test. Being able to carry on a conversation as you walk or exercise without becoming out of breath means you are walking at a good pace.

Target Heart Rate. This measure involves periodically checking your pulse as you exercise and staying within a target heart rate range. If your pulse is below the low end of the range, you need to increase your activity, and if your pulse exceeds the high end of the range, you need to slow down a bit.

If you are exercising to benefit your heart but your pulse rate does not minimally increase, your exercise time is not productive. If your pulse rate exceeds the maximum, it can be dangerous to your heart. Some people assume that the higher they can get their heart to pump, the better. Nothing can be further from the truth. You need to get that heart pumping in your individual target zone.

To find your target heart range, subtract your age from 220 and then multiply by the low and high percentages below.

- Seniors: 50 to 65 percent
- Beginner: 50 to 70 percent
- Regular exerciser: 65 to 80 percent
- Athlete: 75 to 85 percent

Determining the target heart rate for a senior beginning exercise at age 68:

- 220 – 68 = 152.
- 152 x 0.50 = 76 beats per minute (bpm) and 152 x 0.65 = 99 bpm.
- Target range = 76 to 99 bpm.

Example of target heart rate for a beginner at age 55:

- 220 – 55 = 165. 165 x 0.50 = 83 bpm and 165 x 0.70 = 116 bpm
- Target range = 83 to 116 bpm.

Example of target heart rate for a regular exerciser at age 42:

- 220 – 42 = 178. 178 x 0.65 = 116 bpm and 178 x 0.80 = 143 bpm.
- Target range = 116 to 143 bpm.

Target heart rate for an athlete at age 26:

- 220 – 26 = 194. 194 x 0.75 = 146 bpm and 194 x 0.85 = 165 bpm.
- Target range = 146 to 165 bpm.

According to the AHA, when starting an exercise program, aim at the lower percentage of your target zone. Gradually build up to the higher percentage of your target zone.*

---

*When you calculate your target heart rate for cardio-benefit exercise, please confirm it with your physician, who may be aware of other variables that need to be taken into consideration given your health history. Additionally, some high blood pressure medications lower the maximum heart rate and thus the target zone rate. If you're taking such medicine, consult your physician to find out if you need to use a lower target heart rate.

Though it may seem tempting to exceed your target heart range in the hope of speeding up weight loss or getting in shape faster, it is not a good idea. The target heart range is the heart rate at which you are getting cardiovascular and calorie-burning benefits while not overtaxing your heart or respiratory system. Exercising over your target heart rate for a period of time is stressful to the heart and your body and is a risk rather than a benefit.

MONITORING YOUR HEART RATE

One way to monitor your heart rate during exercise is to take your pulse at your wrist or neck. First, measure the number of heartbeats for fifteen seconds, then multiply by four, and that will be your number of beats per minute. So, if I have thirty-five heartbeats in fifteen seconds, that's 140 beats per minute. This is at the high end of a 42-year-old regular exerciser's target range of 116–142.

Some people find it difficult to take their pulse during exercise. An alternative to measuring your own pulse is to purchase a heart rate monitor. Some of these are designed like a wrist watch; others are chest strap units that constantly monitor your heart rate through the chest strap and transmit the reading to a wrist unit for you to check whenever you wish. Some treadmills or elliptical machines have a pulse bar that checks your heart rate any time during your exercise period.

Remember, you should never exercise at 100 percent of your maximal heart rate.

OTHER WAYS TO MOVE YOUR BODY

Old and young alike can benefit from any and all increases in physical activity. The latest research on exercise tells us that older people of all physical conditions have much to gain from exercise and staying physically active. They also have much to lose if they become physically inactive. There are four types of exercise that give different benefits. Every one of them is a plus for those with Met B, prediabetes, and type 2 diabetes:

Aerobic exercises are activities that raise your heart rate and breathing for an extended period of time. The benefits of aerobic-type activity include improving breathing capacity, increasing muscle strength (including heart muscle strength), improving circulation, and increasing endurance. Examples of aerobic exercise include walking, riding a stationary bike or bicycling, swimming, raking leaves, dancing, walking on the treadmill, or using an elliptical machine. Aerobic activity helps lower blood sugar.

Strength exercises are activities that help retain muscle and improve muscle tone to make you stronger. Retaining muscle helps stoke your metabolic rate, aids in weight loss, improves blood sugar, and helps prevent osteoporosis. Strength exercises include light weight training with the use of dumbbells and a bench or the use of a stability ball. You can purchase this basic equipment in any sporting goods department. Gyms have all-in-one machines that provide a workout like weight training with dumbbells.

Balance exercises help prevent falls in older adults. Each year, more than 1.7 million older Americans end up in emergency rooms for injuries due to falls. Balance exercises can build up leg muscles to make you more stable for your everyday tasks. You can do balance exercises anytime and anyplace. If you are unsteady, have a sturdy chair (or person) nearby to assist.

- Walk heel-to-toe. Position your heel just in front of the toes of the opposite foot each time you take a step. Your heel and toes should touch or almost touch as you walk.

- Stand on one foot (while waiting in line at the grocery store or at the bus stop, for example). Alternate feet.
- Stand up and sit down without using your hands.

Stretching exercises give you more freedom of movement, increase flexibility, and allow you to be more limber. Stretching exercises alone will not help with strength or endurance. Tai chi and yoga are examples of stretching exercises.

EXERCISING WITH DIABETES

Having diabetes requires some extra considerations when choosing an exercise regimen, but the many benefits are definitely worth it. As I mentioned, exercise is not an option; it is a necessity. Just about anyone can exercise; even those who are wheelchair-bound or bedridden must move their muscles. "Move them or lose them" are watchwords for those with diabetes. With less muscle tissue, our blood sugar, weight, blood pressure, and mood will suffer.

- Get your physician's approval for exercise if you have been inactive for a period of time. Long-term complications of diabetes, such as damage to the retina, kidneys, heart, or nerves, may need to taken into consideration when determining the type of exercise program that will work for you.
- Wear proper-fitting exercise shoes or sneakers. Some people with diabetes have nerve damage that causes numbness in their feet and toes. As a result, they may not sense irritation, blisters, or inflammation. Always visually inspect your feet when you remove your socks and shoes after your workout. Report any foot problems to your physician.
- Wear 100 percent white cotton socks to allow feet to stay cool and dry.

- If you have a history of eye problems or high blood pressure, weight lifting, calisthenics, or sit-ups may be contraindicated. The ADA discourages power lifting (bench press, dead lift, or squat) for those with moderate retinopathy. Your eye doctor or specialist can answer your questions about weight lifting regarding the condition of your eyes.
- Make sure to drink 8 ounces of water or carb-free fitness water for every thirty minutes of exercise. If you are exercising in hot weather, you might consider upping your water intake to 8 ounces for every fifteen minutes.
- If you are on medication to lower your blood sugar (either oral agents or insulin), always carry a quick source of energy. (I recommend carrying a roll of glucose tablets.) If you are exercising solo, take your glucose tablets, a charged cell phone, personal identification, and water.
- Blood sugar meters are now very portable and fit easily into a jacket, pants, or shorts pocket. Take your meter along if you take insulin or blood sugar lowering medication.
- If you take glucose-lowering medication, consider wearing a medical alert bracelet or necklace. At the very least, put a medical alert card by your license in your wallet. You can also program an "in case of emergency" contact into your phone.
- Walk with a friend. Walking with someone increases your chance of regularly taking that walk, plus there's another person present for safety reasons.
- If you are walking alone, make sure someone knows your usual walk route.
- If there isn't a path or sidewalk and you are walking on the side of the road, walk against oncoming traffic so you can see what or who is coming your way.
- Wear reflective clothing or carry a flashlight if you are walking at night.

- Carry a whistle, pepper spray, or noisemaker in case of an emergency.
- The best time to exercise is one to two hours after eating a meal because the exercise itself will help muscles to burn some of the blood sugar from the meal and less insulin will be required to normalize blood sugar.
- If you are exercising three hours or more after a meal, it is a good idea to have an 11–20 gram carbohydrate snack, such as half a banana, ½ cup natural applesauce, 6 ounces sugar-free yogurt, or 8 ounces nonfat or low-fat milk prior to your exercise.

TESTING YOUR BLOOD SUGAR WHEN YOU EXERCISE AND TAKE MEDICATIONS

If you take insulin or medications that function to lower blood sugar, you should test your blood sugar before exercising. This will determine if your blood sugar is at a safe level to begin exercising and if fueling it forward (see page 176) will be needed during exercise. Remember that your medications and your exercise will lower your blood sugar; failure to fuel appropriately can result in hypoglycemia.

Assessing your pre-exercise blood sugar:

- If blood sugar is **lower than 100 mg/dL**, it may be too low to exercise without fueling it forward (remember that you are taking medication that will continue to lower your blood sugar). You should eat 11–20 grams of carb before you exercise if your blood sugar is under 100 mg/dL. This will fuel your first thirty minutes of activity. If you will exercise more than thirty minutes, take another 11–20 gram carb source at the thirty-minute mark to fuel the upcoming thirty minutes.
- Pre-exercise blood sugar **between 101–180**: There is probably no need to fuel it forward at the start of activity because you may

have enough circulating blood sugar to fuel the first thirty minutes. At the thirty-minute mark, consider fueling the next half hour as directed in fueling it forward guidelines.

- If your blood sugar is **181–280:** There should be no need to fuel it forward; there should be enough fuel to support your workout of up to sixty minutes.
- If your blood sugar is **more than 280:** When blood sugar is this elevated, it may be better to assess the reason for the high reading before you try to lower it through exercise. Drink plenty of water, and don't exert yourself with exercise at this time. If high readings persist, contact your doctor for possible medication intervention. An unexpectedly high blood sugar may indicate that you are sick or getting sick, have an infection, are responding to high stress, may have forgotten to take blood sugar–lowering medications, or are reacting to pain.

TREATING HYPOGLYCEMIA

If you take medication to lower blood sugar and feel any symptoms of hypoglycemia* while exercising, you should:

- Stop exercising immediately
- If you have your meter, check your blood sugar and treat the hypoglycemia if the reading is under 70 mg/dL
- If you have no meter and you feel dizzy, shaky, anxious, or confused, stop exercising and treat the hypoglycemia

---

*Those who take medication to lower blood sugar may become hypoglycemic during or hours after exercise. The symptoms may include dizziness, light-headedness, blurry vision, inability to speak coherently, nausea, feeling of "emptiness," strong need for carbohydrate, rapid heartbeat, cold sweats, irritability, and anxiety.

To treat the hypoglycemia, if blood sugar is 50–70 mg/dL, choose one of the following:
- 3–4 glucose tabs
- ½ cup fruit juice (or 4 ounce juice box)
- ½ can regular soda (6 ounces)
- 3 packets of sugar
- 1 tablespoon honey

To treat hypoglycemia if blood sugar is under 50 mg/dL, you will initially double the treatment:
- 6–8 glucose tablets
- 8 ounces juice
- 12 ounces regular soda
- 6 packets sugar
- 2 tablespoons honey

Recheck your blood sugar ten minutes later. If blood sugar remains under 80 mg/dL, repeat single treatment and retest ten minutes later. Repeat treatment as needed until blood sugar reaches at least 80 mg/dL (3.9 mmol/L).* See Chapter 14 for more details about treating hypoglycemia.

FREQUENTLY ASKED QUESTIONS ABOUT EXERCISE

I don't take medication for diabetes. Will I become hypoglycemic (low blood sugar reaction) if I exercise and have Met B, prediabetes, or diabetes?

---

*If you have treated low blood sugar three times in thirty minutes, and it has not reached a minimum of 80, seek medical attention.

It is uncommon for hypoglycemia to occur when you have Met B, prediabetes, or diabetes and take no medication to lower blood sugar.

Exercise always drops blood sugar, right?

Oddly enough, blood sugar can rise or fall during and after exercise. An easy way to monitor the direction of your blood sugar is to get a reading before, during (if you feel hypoglycemic), and after exercise. (Blood sugar can drop hours after you exercise because your muscles continue to uptake blood sugar from your bloodstream.) If you take no medication for diabetes, you will most likely not experience low blood sugar, but if you do take medication to lower blood sugar (insulin or certain oral medications), you should test your blood sugar before, during if you feel low, and after to make sure you are safe to drive.

For those with Met B, prediabetes, or type 2 diabetes, a combination of diet (Steps 1, 2, or 3 of the Diabetes Miracle) plus regular physical activity is the one-two punch required to knock out uncontrolled blood sugar and improve your overall metabolism, help you reach and maintain your desired weight, maintain great health, and foster lifelong well-being. Combine the right diet with regular exercise, and watch what happens!

MONITORING YOUR BLOOD SUGAR

Checking your own blood sugar is one of the best ways to know how well your diabetes treatment plan is working on a daily basis and to provide real-time information to your physician as she makes important decisions regarding medications and doses—or even the elimination of medications.

If you are worried that checking your blood sugar will be painful, you can breathe a sigh of relief. Today's monitoring methods have come a long way since our grandparents' or parents' days. Not so many years ago, there were no machines to read blood sugar samples. People had to stick their fingers without the benefit of a lancing device and obtain a large sample of blood to cover an area on a test strip. After exactly the right amount of time, the blood was wiped off and a color change on the strip was compared to a color chart on the strip bottle. By guesstimating the color of the strip (everyone has his own color perception), blood sugar range was estimated.

Because a large drop of blood was required, the finger-stick required a thick lancet and was deep and quite painful. The monitoring process took time, it was messy, and blood sugar testing was not very accurate. But back in the day, there was no other way.

Many people remember their parents and grandparents performing antiquated blood sugar self-monitoring and want no part of it in their own lives. These people may not realize that technological strides have replaced the barbaric methods used just twenty-five years ago. Today's blood glucose–monitoring devices are now smaller than a cell phone, use very fine lancets that have adjustable depth settings, and provide surprisingly accurate information in a matter of seconds.

Another reason why people might forgo self-monitoring of blood sugar is because they believe that they know what their sugar is reading at any given time. Truth be known, unless your blood sugar drops below 65 or exceeds 200 mg/dL, you probably won't experience symptoms. People can live for years with elevated blood sugar without feeling traditional symptoms, but this does not mean that elevated blood sugar is meaningless or harmless. Even a person who has had diabetes for many years cannot accurately predict blood sugar, and some people with dangerously high blood sugar for a period of years have become accustomed to what those high readings feel like. The high readings have become their norm.

Keep in mind that blood sugar spikes of more than 140 mg/dL can begin to chip away at your body's health. Long-term mild elevations (even without symptoms) can cause the same complications as high readings cause over a shorter period of time. This is why it is important not to wait to feel sick from diabetes to start to control diabetes.

I have had type 2 diabetes for almost fifteen years and have worked as a diabetes nutritionist and educator, spending each and every day immersed in the field of diabetes for more than thirty years. Even with all this exposure to diabetes and with my own blood sugar issues, I cannot accurately predict my blood glucose at any given time. I test my blood sugar twice a day, every day, to make certain that I am in the driver's seat with my diabetes.

TESTING 1, 2, 3

Mario was diagnosed with type 2 diabetes when he was 58 years old. He had always been a proud man, very macho, and had a tough demeanor. Only his diabetes educator knew that he was afraid to test his blood sugar because he hated needles.

I told Mario a needle isn't used to test blood sugar; rather, it is a lancet. A needle (what he visualized as part of a syringe) is usually used to inject or withdraw something from the body. We use needles to administer insulin and also to obtain a blood sample at the lab.

A lancet makes a tiny prick to obtain a tiny blood droplet. Mario didn't want to hear about it. "I remember watching my Nona stick her finger. She always made a noise and jumped, and the blood drop looked very large."

I explained to Mario that things have changed. The sample of blood needed is about the size of a pencil point, so the lancet does not have to go deeply into the finger. There are lancing devices that can be set to minimize the depth of the finger-prick, and the strips themselves wick the blood sample off of the finger.

I told Mario a few techniques for easily obtaining a blood sample: (1) wash his hands with soap and warm water and rinse with warm water prior to testing; (2) warm his hand prior to obtaining a sample to help dilate blood vessels and bring blood to the surface; (3) shake the hand as if he were shaking down a thermometer to help bring blood closer to the fingertip's surface; (4) test on the outer sides of the index or middle finger, in the area of the cushiony pad of the fingertip because this area has fewer nerve endings than the center of the fingertip; and (5) steady the finger against a tabletop or counter to give support (this strategy also keeps the height of the finger lower than the height of the heart, which helps blood flow more easily).

I also told him that although it is possible to use a lancet more than once (as long as you wash your hands and are the only person using the lancing device), a brand new lancet for every test is the most pain-free way to go, as with each use, the lancet becomes duller.

About two weeks later, I got an email from Mario. It made me smile. He said it took him over a week to get up the nerve to test. He followed the guidelines, did the test, and was shocked when he saw a droplet of blood appear on his finger.

He had been testing ever since and was emailing in his readings. From his results, we could see that his blood sugar was normal, and he noted that he felt good about seeing results as they occurred. He was back in control—and Mario liked being in control.

Painful Finger-Sticks?

You have probably seen advertisements for home glucose monitors that claim to "eliminate the need for painful finger-sticks." The company fails to mention that their monitoring system still requires the use of a lancet, a lancing device, and a tiny drop of blood. They sidestep the fact that their product requires a stick from a site other than your finger.

Keep in mind that when blood sugar is rising or falling rapidly, off-site testing (testing from a site other than the fingertip) is not as reliable or accurate as a finger-stick. There is ongoing work to develop an alternate method of blood glucose measurement that does not require a blood sample. I'm sure this technology will exist in the future.

MONITORING BLOOD SUGAR PROVIDES REAL-TIME RESULTS

If you have diabetes, you can play an important role in your own medical care. Type 2 diabetes can be controlled with lifestyle changes involving diet, exercise, and if necessary medication.

The main goal of management is to keep blood sugar levels within normal or near-normal range with as little medication as necessary. If your body consistently experiences normal blood sugar readings, the complications that would result from years of out of control readings will not occur.

People who experience mostly high readings over a period of time inadvertently set the bar for their body to tolerate blood sugar in excess of what is normal. The person gradually becomes accustomed to how high readings make her feel. Ironically, when the person starts to make progress in normalizing high readings, she may actually believe she is having a low blood sugar reaction.

IS IT HYPOGLYCEMIA?

If you are starting the Diabetes Miracle program with an A1C of 7.5 or higher, you might initially feel a bit fatigued, dizzy, light-headed, and shaky as your blood sugar returns to a normal range. Instead of assuming that you are hypoglycemic based on these symptoms, it would be prudent to check your blood sugar at that time. If the reading is under 70, you are experiencing hypoglycemia (see Chapter 14 for hypoglycemia treatment). If, however, you find your reading is in the normal range, don't treat it as hypoglycemia. Treating a 100 mg/dL blood sugar with four glucose tabs will pop your sugar back into an unhealthy range. Your body may temporarily feel better (because it is accustomed to 160 blood sugar), but you will have taken steps backward in normalizing blood sugar.*

BLOOD SUGAR GOALS FOR HOME MONITORING WHEN YOU HAVE DIABETES

The ADA recommends normal or near-normal blood sugar levels and defines tight control as:

- Fasting or pre-meal blood sugar: 70–130 mg/dL (3.89–7.22 mmol/L)
- Two hours after start of a meal: 180 mg/dL or less (10.00 mmol/L)
- Hemoglobin A1C under 7 percent.

I believe that the ADA guidelines are too liberal for long-term blood glucose control and prefer to use American Association of Clinical Endocrinologists (AACE) guidelines for long-term health and decreased risk of diabetes complications. The 2007 guidelines of the AACE

---

*If you are driving or operating machinery when you feel hypoglycemic, always treat the feeling as if it IS hypoglycemia. You can't afford to assume your sugar is normalizing when it may indeed be hypoglycemia. Low blood sugar can cause dizziness, impaired reaction time, poor judgment, and blurred vision, all symptoms that should never occur while driving or operating machinery.

"encourage patients to achieve blood sugar levels as near normal as possible without inducing low blood sugar (hypoglycemia)":

- Fasting blood sugar: 110 mg/dL or less (6.11 mmol/L)
- Two hours after the start of a meal: 140 mg/dL or less (7.78 mmol/L)
- Hemoglobin A1C: less than 6.5 percent.

Your physician will work with you to establish your target blood glucose range.

PREVENTING COMPLICATIONS

Research studies have shown that control of blood glucose, blood pressure, and blood lipid levels helps prevent complications in people with type 1 or type 2 diabetes.

In 1993, after a ten-year comprehensive study of blood sugar control and outcomes on more than 1,400 people with type 1 diabetes, the results of the Diabetes Control and Complications Trial (DCCT) concluded that when blood sugar was kept as close to normal as possible, study participants had a significantly lower chance of developing complications to the eye, kidney, and nerves.* The most significant of the DCCT findings are as follows:

- 76 percent reduced risk for eye disease with tight control of glucose
- 50 percent reduced risk for kidney disease with tight control of glucose
- 60 percent reduced risk for nerve disease with tight control of glucose.

---

*New England Journal of Medicine 329, no. 14 (September 30, 1993).

When the DCCT study ended, researchers continued to study more than 90 percent of the participants. The follow-up study was called the Epidemiology of Diabetes Interventions and Complications (EDIC).* It assessed the incidence of cardiovascular events, such as heart attack, stroke, or the need for heart surgery, as well as the complications related to the eye, kidney, and nerves. This time around, the study was also examining the impact of intense control to quality of life and cost-effectiveness. EDIC findings confirmed that intense glucose control reduces risk of cardiovascular disease by 42 percent and that of nonfatal heart attack, stroke, or death from cardiovascular causes by 57 percent.

WHAT THE RESULTS OF THE DCCT AND EDIC STUDIES MEAN FOR PEOPLE WITH TYPE 2 DIABETES

The microvascular (small blood vessel) disease development that affects the eye, kidney, nerves, and cardiovascular system is likely similar for both type 1 and type 2 diabetes. In 1998, the United Kingdom Prospective Diabetes Study (UKPDS) identified the importance of good glucose control and blood pressure in the delay or progression of the complications of type 2 diabetes.

Research studies have shown that control of blood glucose, blood pressure, and blood lipid levels helps prevent complications in people with type 1 or type 2 diabetes.

New England Journal of Medicine 353, no. 25 (December 22, 2005).

A New Measure—
Estimated Average Glucose (eAG)

A common complaint that I hear about HbA1C is that the results are given as a percentage. People who monitor their blood sugar are accustomed to addressing their blood sugar as a number in mg/dL, such as 130 mg/dL or 95 mg/dL. A large international study[*] established that A1C is a valid measure of average blood glucose. However, this study sought a way to make the results fall in line with the way people relate to their blood sugar in home monitoring terms.

The A1C-derived average glucose (ADAG) study sought to develop a table of estimated average glucose values that correspond to A1C results. So, instead of just seeing 6.0 percent as your A1C, you'll also get an eAG of 126, which will be more familiar, based on the readings your see every day on your meter.

What if the numbers you've seen on your meter are all in the 90–130 range, but your eAG is 154? Well, you might only be testing first thing in the morning, and your readings may very well be 90–130 in the morning. The eAG will pick up all your readings, 24 hours a day, two to three months back. You definitely are spiking regularly somewhere during the day. Maybe it would be a good idea to check your blood sugar two hours after your largest meal or in the middle of the night and see what your meter shows at alternate times of day or night.

[*]A1C-Derived Average Glucose Study. Available at www.ncbi.nlm.nih.gov/pubmed/19012527.

HERE'S HOW THE A1C RELATES TO THE NEW EAG*

A1C (%)	eAG (mg/dL)
5.0	97
5.5	111
6.0	126
6.5	140
7.0	154
7.5	169
8.0	183
8.5	197
9.0	212
9.5	226
10.0	240
10.5	255
11.0	269
11.5	283
12.0	298

MONITORING YOUR BLOOD SUGAR

If your physician recommends blood sugar monitoring, or if you have a diagnosis of prediabetes or type 2 diabetes and you would like to test your blood sugar, ask your doctor for a prescription that reads: "Blood glucose monitor, blood glucose testing lancets, blood glucose test strips."

Obtaining a Blood Glucose Meter. You can purchase a blood glucose meter, strips, and lancets without a prescription at a local pharmacy, supermarket, or chain superstore. However, you may wish to obtain one with a prescription because some insurance companies cover some portion of the cost of the meter and monitoring supplies. Do ask a certified diabetes educator, physician, or endocrinologist for their recommendation for a preferred meter brand.

---

*American Diabetes Association, "Estimated Average Glucose," http://professional
.diabetes.org/glucosecalculator.aspx. Accessed April 2009.

Most people with type 2 diabetes who use insulin obtain a prescription to test up to six times a day. Most people with type 2 diabetes not using insulin obtain a prescription for three to four tests a day. You may not need to test this often, but just in case, you will have adequate supplies.

HOW TO USE A BLOOD GLUCOSE METER

Your blood sugar monitor will come with an instruction guide and may contain a "Quick and Easy" one-page set of instructions. The meter company's website most likely also provides a video demonstration of its monitor's use. You can use the 24/7 hotline number provided by your meter company: The technical support is usually very good. (The 800 number is usually on the back of the meter itself.) Here are the basic instructions:

1. Always wash your hands with soap and warm water before testing. If you are not near a sink, use an alcohol wipe to cleanse the finger tip. In either case, dry your hands thoroughly before obtaining your blood sample.
2. Insert a new lancet into the lancing device. Although some people re-use their personal lancets, they do dull with repeated use and become more painful.
3. Insert the test strip into the monitor as directed by the instructions. Some monitors require coding the machine to match the code on the test strip vial, whereas other strips require no coding.
4. Use the lancing device to obtain a small drop of blood from your fingertip. I prefer not to prick the tip of my fingertip because it is more sensitive. If you place the lancing device slightly off center on the fatty pad of the finger, it is less sensitive. (There is usually a depth setting on the lancing device. Most people use the lowest

number that allows them to obtain an adequate sample. The higher the depth setting, the deeper the puncture. (I use setting 1 or 2.)

5. People who are right-handed usually hold the lancing device in their right hand and test a finger on their left hand, and vice versa.

6. If you have difficulty getting enough blood from the fingertip, try rinsing your fingers again with warm water (dry them after), shake your hand below waist level, or gently squeeze the fingertip.

7. Apply the blood drop to the test strip in the blood glucose meter. The results will be displayed on the meter after several seconds.

8. Dispose of the used lancet in a puncture-resistant sharps container (not in household trash). The strip can be disposed of in the regular trash.

9. Although most meters have a built-in memory to store readings, many people use a computer program (accessed through the meter company) that places readings in a virtual blood sugar log and can print graphs and charts to show your personal blood sugar trends. You might also choose to handwrite your results in the log book that comes with your meter. The log book gives a clear visual reference of the patterns of blood sugar at certain times and allows you to see in an instant your personal blood glucose trends, such as high readings after dinner or normal readings in the morning.*

The results on a home glucose monitor are not an exact match to the results obtained through a venous blood draw in a lab. For the time being, they are the best results that can be obtained for home use (in five seconds!). However, diabetes should not be diagnosed from a result on a home glucose monitor.

---

*See log book samples on pages 341–343.

BEST TIMES FOR TESTING

Your physician should give you directions as to how often and when to test your blood sugar based on your treatment plan for diabetes. The following is a guideline only.

Fasting means first thing when you wake up for the day, as soon as possible. The longer you wait to test, even though you haven't eaten yet, the higher your reading may rise because of liver sugar release.

Two-hour after readings are taken two hours after the START of a meal.

Type 2 diabetes treated with diet and exercise (no meds) = test two to four times/day: fasting and two hours after a meal.

Type 2 diabetes treated with diet, exercise, and oral meds = test two to four times a day: fasting and two hours after a meal or if you are feeling hypoglycemic.

Type 2 diabetes treated with diet, exercise, and insulin = test four to six times a day: fasting, before lunch, dinner, bedtime, and if you are feeling hypoglycemic.

GOALS FOR FASTING BLOOD GLUCOSE HOME MONITORING READINGS

Consider the following reasonable goals for home monitoring for fasting readings:

- For those with Met B: fasting blood glucose 100 or less
- AACE: Those with type 2 diabetes: fasting glucose 110 or less
- ADA: Those with type 2 diabetes: fasting glucose 130 or less

Your fasting blood glucose reading has little to do with what you ate for dinner the night before. When a person wakes up with a 165 mg/dL blood sugar result, she often thinks back to what she ate at dinner the previous night or blames her nighttime snack for the high reading.

Fasting blood sugar primarily reflects the glycogen released by the liver while you sleep. Whenever you go for more than five hours without eating, your liver automatically deposits fuel into your bloodstream in the form of blood sugar. So, if you had dinner at 7:00 PM and consumed no nighttime snack, your liver would release sugar at about midnight and again at about 5:00 AM. When you wake up at 6:30 AM and check your sugar, the reading you see reflects the sugar that has been released from the liver, not what you ate twelve hours before.

IF YOUR FASTING NUMBER IS ELEVATED

Many people believe that when their fasting reading is elevated, they should skip or delay breakfast, believing that more food will cause the already elevated reading to rise even higher. Ironically, the longer you wait to eat after waking up, the higher the reading will rise (because of more liver glycogen involvement). Using the previous scenario, your liver released glycogen at 12:00 AM and 5:00 AM. At 6:30, you tested and saw a 165. If you think, "I'm going to wait until the reading drops before I eat," your liver will once again release glycogen at 10:00 AM. So delaying or skipping breakfast is not the answer.

If you have diabetes and on occasion your fasting blood sugar exceeds 120, drink a tall glass of water and eat your appropriate breakfast or a snack. The action of eating will put you, not your liver, in the driver's seat.

CONSISTENTLY HIGH FASTING LEVELS

If your fasting blood sugar is consistently elevated, your physician may want to prescribe medication to bring the readings into the normal range. Remember that this medication is not treating the root of the problem; it is band-aiding the effect of the problem and enabling your reading to land in the normal range.

Before medication is initiated, it might be prudent to try the following nonmedicinal ways to decrease fasting readings.

- Have an appropriate snack within an hour of bedtime and again in the middle of the night. This action is intended to decrease the number and amount of nighttime glycogen releases from the liver.
- Test your blood sugar as soon as you wake up. The longer you wait to test, the higher the reading will be. Plan to have a snack or breakfast within one hour of rising.
- To facilitate better wake-up readings, do some of your physical activity after dinner. Exercise done about one to two hours after your dinner helps lower your post-dinner blood sugar reading and will improve your next morning's fasting reading. Exercise enables muscles to uptake blood sugar for hours after the activity ends, so the exercise you do at 8:00 PM can help lower your blood sugar into the next morning.
- Fasting readings can rise from stress, pain, illness, or certain medications. Sometimes you need to treat the pain, constructively deal with stress, get well, review any medications you are taking to see if they impact blood sugar, or ask your physician about a temporary medication to help the fasting reading until you get the stressor under control.

If you are in chronic pain and don't treat it, the pain can cause blood sugar readings to rise and might necessitate the need for medication. If your pain is properly managed, you may not need medication for diabetes.

If you have tried all the nonmedicinal ways to lower your fasting reading and it remains elevated, you may want to talk to your physician about medication in addition to diet and exercise.

GOALS FOR POST-MEAL BLOOD GLUCOSE HOME MONITORING READINGS

The best time to test your body's reaction to a meal is two hours after the start of a meal. You can choose any meal and check a different meal every day if you want to. If you miss the two-hour mark, you can still test afterward. Just make a note as to how many hours passed from the start of the meal so that reading is analyzed in relation to the meal time.

Consider the following reasonable blood sugar readings for post-meal readings:

- 2 hours after the start of a meal = goal of 140 or less
- 3 hours after the start of a meal = goal of 130 or less
- 4 hours after the start of a meal = goal of 120 or less
- 5 hours after the start of a meal = don't bother testing as you need to eat—your liver is poised to release.

IF POST-MEAL READINGS ARE TOO HIGH

Unlike elevated fasting blood glucose readings, high post-meal readings do *not* indicate that you should eat ASAP. The reading is most likely elevated because of food choices you made at the meal you are testing.

If your post-meal reading is elevated, drink a tall glass of water and get ten or more minutes of physical activity: a brisk ten-minute walk around the building, around your block, up and down the stairs. Or you can lift some light weights. Move your muscles to uptake excess sugar from the bloodstream. You can actually normalize a mildly elevated post-meal reading with a few minutes of exercise.

FASTING AND POST-MEAL TESTING SHOWS TWO DIFFERENT CAUSES OF HIGH BLOOD SUGAR

Your fasting reading has little to do with excess carb consumption from the previous night. If you only tested your blood sugar in the morning, even if you performed this test every day, you would mainly be testing your insulin's response to the liver release of glycogen. This reading is helpful, but it is not the whole picture. Many of my patients had only been testing their blood sugar in the morning for years and never understood why there was such a disparity between their HbA1C and daily fasting readings. They didn't realize that their food-related blood glucose is totally separate from the morning reading, and they were unaware that they were not able to handle the carb at their meal.

IF POST-MEAL READINGS ARE CONSISTENTLY ELEVATED

If your post-meal reading is elevated, this shows that your body is not tolerating the carbohydrate from the meal you just consumed. Don't relate the reading to the portion size of the steak or pieces of chicken or veggies you consumed; think about the amount and type of carbohydrate. Did you consume the correct amount of carbohydrate that matches the step of the Diabetes Miracle you are following?

Before opting for medication, see if the following nonmedicinal tips help bring your after meal readings into normal range:

- Make sure that your carbohydrate intake at meals is within the target range for the step that you are currently following. Make a note next to the high reading if you were off with carb intake. If you can find the reason for your readings being elevated and remedy it, you will not require medication.
- Make sure that you are not allowing five hours to pass without eating. If you delayed your meal, your liver released glycogen at the five-hour mark (without your awareness), and then you ate your "late" meal, the combination of the sugar from the liver and the sugar from the carbohydrate would piggyback to produce a high post-meal reading. Make a notation next to the high reading if you missed your necessary between-meal carb snack.

- Consider physical activity in the morning, one to two hours after breakfast, to help readings after meals for the rest of the day. As previously noted, physical activity helps control blood sugar for hours after the activity. If you exercise after breakfast by taking a brisk walk, you will help blood glucose control until after dinner. All of your post-meal readings can improve from after-breakfast exercise. If you take another walk after dinner at 7:00 PM, your blood sugar will have help until into the morning. By breaking your daily walking into two sessions, you can help improve your blood sugar twenty-four hours a day.

If you have tried all the nonmedicinal ways to lower your post-meal readings and they remain elevated (over 140 at the two-hour mark), it may be time to discuss medication with your doctor.

Other Non Food Reasons for a Blood Sugar Spike

Aside from being affected by food intake and exercise, both fasting and post-meal readings can increase from stress, illness, pain, or certain medications. If you treat the cause of the pain, stress, or illness, all of your readings may improve.

Stress. Stress (emotional or physical) triggers the natural release of stress hormones such as cortisol, adrenaline, or epinephrine. These hormones cause blood sugar to rise for the "fight-or-flight" response to the stress. It is the rise in stress hormone levels and subsequent deluge of liver glycogen that provides the energy to "run from the bad guy."

We all know that much of our stress doesn't involve running from the stressor. We are stressed at home, in our cars, at our jobs, in our families, and so on. The body's reaction to these stressors is the same as if you needed to get out of the way of a speeding train. The abrupt rise in stress hormones causes an abrupt rise in blood sugar.

Certain events in a person's life are naturally stressful: starting a new job, marriage, divorce, adjustment to parenthood, death of a loved one, a car accident, family problems, or financial distress. The natural stress response will trigger high blood sugar readings.

If you are living your healthy lifestyle during stressful times and your blood sugar is elevated because of stress, you may temporarily require medication. When the stress abates, your physician can reevaluate the need for medication.

Illness. Illness is considered a stress to the body and can also lead to the need for medication. Many people who normally take oral medication for diabetes require insulin when they are hospitalized. After discharge, when they are on the mend, they can usually revert back to oral medication. Certain medications themselves cause blood sugar to rise. Steroid-based medications (cortisone, prednisone) increase blood sugar. Oftentimes, increased dosages of diabetes medication are needed when a steroidal medication is required. When the treatment ends, it is possible that medication will return to normal doses.

Pain. Pain is another stressor that causes the release of stress hormones. If a patient is in chronic pain, he may require medication to help control blood sugar. If the pain is caused by an acute injury, it is probable that medication needs will revert to normal when the pain subsides.

Inactivity. Certain life situations can temporarily or permanently decrease a person's ability to get adequate physical activity. If a person is unable to move or perform her normal physical activity, blood sugar will rise, and medication may temporarily be needed until she is able to move again. If a person is chronically immobilized, it would be helpful to ask for a physical therapy review to determine if less conventional types of exercise may be considered. Any exercise is better than no exercise when it comes to diabetes. The less physical activity a person gets, the more medication he will require—and every medication has side effects.

Two Machines; Two Different Readings

The gold standard for measuring glucose is a large chemistry analyzer in a lab, which measures glucose values in plasma obtained from a blood vessel with a needle. The diagnosis of diabetes should be made from a venous blood draw (lab drawn, not home monitoring). The blood obtained from a finger-prick for home glucose monitoring is capillary whole blood. It typically gives a different value. As of 2011, the majority of home glucose monitors are calibrated so as to be comparable to venous plasma glucose readings. Read your monitor's paperwork to find out about your device.

Portable finger-stick glucose meters are not as accurate as you might expect. From one meter to another, blood sugar may vary by as much as 20 percent. If your actual glucose level is 100 mg/dL, the meter may report it as 80 or 120 or anywhere in between. The meters tend to be less accurate at glucose values of more than 200 mg/dL. Some devices tend to be more accurate than others. Your endocrinologist or diabetes educator can advise you on the monitors she has found to be most accurate when compared to a venous blood test.

WHEN YOU GET A VERY HIGH READING

As a person with type 2 diabetes, I am well aware that it is impossible to always have perfectly normal blood sugar. Many outside influences can pop your number higher than usual, including stress, pain, illness, hormonal changes during the menstrual cycle, lack of exercise, and dietary issues. Whenever a reading is elevated above what I feel it should be given my diet and exercise, I always try to determine what could have caused it and make a tiny notation in my blood sugar log next to the number (stress, pain, lack of exercise) so I can pinpoint what my current lifestyle stressors are and work on resolving them.

There have been a few times in my life when my home meter registered a reading considerably out of the normal range. Instead of panicking that I was in major trouble, I needed to find out if the reading was accurate. Each monitor has its own control solution, and each vial of test strips is stamped with a control range. The control solution is a liquid sugar solution, and the control range is the range that the sugar solution will register if the strip and the machine are in proper order. Some new meters come packed with this tiny vial of control solution; others require that you purchase control solution from the company. (Once you open the control solution's seal, it is viable for three months.)

Let's say that I checked my blood sugar two hours after dinner and it registered 270 mg/dL instead of its usual 120–130. I know that I ate correctly, am experiencing no major stress, am not sick, and have no pain—but my reading is off the charts. I have to question the accuracy of the test.

I generally rewash my hands and test again because it might have been one rogue test strip that read incorrectly. I have also known patients who have skewed their readings with hand lotions or the remnants of an orange's juice.

If after retesting you get another sky-high reading for no apparent reason, you can check the machine itself: Shake the bottle of control solution, apply a drop to your finger, and perform a test using the control as your sample. If the meter and strip are working properly, the reading will fall within the control range on the strip's vial. This will attest that your blood sugar is, indeed, in the range the meter showed.

If you can pinpoint the cause of the high reading, you can easily correct it. If, however, you analyze your life and can't find the reason that your readings are elevated, don't hesitate to call your physician's office to report these off-the-wall readings. If readings remain elevated for no apparent reason, it may be time for a medication change or increase.

MY FASTING BLOOD GLUCOSE LEVELS

When I am using a home monitor, I strive to keep my fasting blood glucose under 120 mg/dL. As I do not currently take medication to lower blood sugar, I will allow my fasting number to be as high as 120 mg/dL in the morning. I also check my blood sugar two hours after my largest meal of the day and work to keep readings under 140 mg/dL. I am currently able to maintain these readings taking no medication for diabetes. If I were to take medication for diabetes, I can easily "create" a fasting reading under 100 mg/dL—but I choose not to take medication as long as my readings remain "normal" for me.

After weighing the risk and benefit of taking a medication to force a morning reading under 100 or living long-term with a fasting number under 120, I have opted for the under-120 fasting number and under-140 postprandial readings with lifestyle modifications only. You can consult with your physician to decide what readings make the most sense for you on a long-term basis. Every medication has a side effect, and the less medication you can take and still safeguard your health, the better.

My diagnosis of diabetes has had a positive effect on my life. It gives me a daily incentive to eat right, exercise, drink more water, take my multivitamins/supplements, spread out my eating throughout the day, reduce stress, and get adequate sleep—all things that everyone should do to maintain a healthy body.

FREQUENTLY ASKED QUESTIONS

Why do I need a hemoglobin A1C test when I check my blood sugar at home twice a day every day?

The results of home glucose monitoring or a fasting blood sugar lab test reflect your blood sugar at that moment in time. Blood sugar peaks and valleys occur all day and night, every day and night. These all-day occurrences are not reflected in the results of a self-test. The HbA1C test looks at the average of highs and lows around the clock, for the last two to three months in time, and gives you an idea of your overall blood sugar control.

The complications of diabetes occur over time from excess blood sugar that candy-coats proteins in the body. (See complications, pages 100–111.) HbA1C is a good indicator of what is happening in other tissues of the body. High A1C readings mean you are at greater risk for diabetes complications. Conversely, normal A1C levels are associated with a lower risk of complications.

Studies have shown that for every 1 percent drop in HbA1C, the risk of microvascular complications is decreased by 10 percent. If a person starts out with a 9 percent A1C and makes changes necessary to decrease A1C to 6 percent, he can consider that he decreased his risk of microvascular complications by about 30 percent. Consider this: Uncontrolled type 2 diabetes has the ability to cause health problems with your eyes, nerves, blood vessels, circulation, kidneys, and more . . . but type 2 diabetes is controllable. Tracking A1C keeps tabs on where you stand regarding 24/7 control.

Why should I bother testing my blood sugar daily when I have my hemoglobin A1C checked several times a year at my physician's office?

Blood sugar can rise quietly and unnoticeably: a high reading here, a high reading there, high readings in the middle of the night, high readings that occur when you are overly stressed or sick. If you notice that your A1C is 6.1 in January but 7.1 in May, you know that your average blood sugar is trending up, significantly. You do not, however, know when during the day/night your levels are high.

If your HbA1C blood test is rising despite positive changes you make to help lower it (diet, exercise, and stress reduction), you may need to discuss with your doctor the use of medication to lower your blood sugar. Remember that the A1C test does not pinpoint when you are having a problem. You can use home glucose monitoring to pinpoint the problem areas in the day and focus your attention on improving them. Certain medications correct high fasting readings; others help lower post-meal readings. For these reasons, it is important to perform daily home glucose monitoring AND have A1C checked at your physician visits (quarterly is recommended).

HANDLING HYPOGLYCEMIA

Most people think the complications of diabetes are only caused by high blood sugar. But, the complication I'd like to discuss involves low blood sugar.

Blood sugar less than 70 mg/dL is considered hypoglycemia (low blood sugar), although symptoms are not usually apparent until blood sugar drops below 65 mg/dL. As sugar drops below 70 mg/dL, the brain initially sends signals to the person to eat carbohydrates to lift the blood glucose. Blood sugar less than 70 can begin to trigger hypoglycemia's symptoms, which include:

- light-headedness
- hunger
- weakness
- cold sweat
- shakiness
- irritability
- palpitations
- difficulty speaking.

If the person fails to eat in answer to the brain's "call to sugar," the next step is the release of hormones, including glucagon, cortisol, and epinephrine—with the intent of forcing blood sugar to rise. These hormones trigger an immediate release of sugar from the liver's glycogen stores.

As hypoglycemia evolves, the brain becomes starved for fuel and triggers hunger or requests immediate sugar release from liver stores as a built-in survival mechanism. The brain is the main organ affected by low blood glucose because it cannot makes its own sugar, and glucose is its preferred energy source. Only if absolutely necessary, and very reluctantly, the brain can utilize ketones (fat) as fuel.

It is unusual for blood sugar to drop below 65 mg/dL without the body's natural hunger and hormonal mechanism kicking in to automatically raise blood sugar levels back into the normal range. A problem can arise when a person with diabetes takes glucose-lowering medication (either oral medications or insulin). If medication-taking diabetics fail to eat in a timely manner, skip meals, or exercise for a prolonged period of time without eating, they run the risk of medication-induced low blood sugar, which requires immediate treatment. The medications can override the liver's ability to raise blood sugar, and blood sugar might continue to drop to a dangerous level.

If a person is experiencing hypoglycemia, the treatment involves a quick-acting source of easily absorbed carbohydrate. It takes about ten minutes for the hypoglycemic treatment to take effect. (See treatment of hypoglycemia on pages 294–295.)

Note that ice cream, cake, and chocolate should not be used to treat hypoglycemia. The carb source should not contain fat or protein because this will slow its absorption. Use approximately 15 grams of rapid-acting carbohydrate for the best results.

WHEN HYPOGLYCEMIA REQUIRES EMERGENCY TREATMENT

If the hypoglycemic episode has progressed to the point that the person cannot or will not take anything by mouth or is unconscious, more drastic measures will be needed. As time is of the essence, first call 911.

An injection of glucagon (a prescription version of the liver hormone), given into a muscle, will cause the liver to rapidly release sugar stores. The effect takes but a few minutes and lasts for about sixty to ninety minutes. Once blood sugar has risen to the normal range, a source of carb and protein should be given as a snack or meal. It is a good idea for family members or roommates of insulin-requiring patients to be trained in glucagon injections.

If a glucagon pen is not available and the patient cannot take carbohydrate by mouth, emergency responders will either administer glucagon or start IV glucose. A person with a history of low blood glucose reactions should report them to her physician because a change in medication type or dosage is required. Repeated bouts of hypoglycemia are not normal, and changes must be made to prevent them from happening.

AVOIDING HYPOGLYCEMIA

In order to avoid having a hypoglycemia emergency, do the following:

1. Eat! Oftentimes the onset of hypoglycemia is from skipping meals when insulin or medication for diabetes has been taken. If you are on glucose-lowering medication, you cannot skip a meal.
2. Monitor your intake of alcoholic beverages in relation to your medication and meals. Alcohol can temporarily suppress the liver from releasing glucose. If you've had a drink or two, you may actually precipitate hypoglycemia.

3. If you are on blood glucose–lowering medication, you may need to check blood sugar before and after exercise as well as later in the day. Muscles will uptake sugar for hours after exercise is concluded.*

HYPOGLYCEMIC UNAWARENESS

A person who has struggled with repeated low blood sugar reactions over a period of time may develop hypoglycemic unawareness: The body becomes so accustomed to low blood sugar that it no longer registers the warning signals of hypoglycemia until the readings become very low. Stabilizing and normalizing blood sugar—in effect, prohibiting the lows—will help to bring back a person's awareness of hypoglycemia.

Conversely, a person who has been living with high blood sugar for a period of time may experience all the symptoms of low blood sugar as their blood sugar returns from high levels into the normal range. They may feel as if their blood sugar is 65 when it is in fact 125. If they automatically treat the normal 125 as a low blood sugar, they will pop their sugar back into the unhealthy high range and never adjust to normal blood sugar. When a person with diabetes alters diet or exercise regimens, changes medication type, or changes medication dosages, more frequent blood sugar testing may be required temporarily to ascertain blood sugar response.

A MEASURED RESPONSE TO HYPOGLYCEMIA

The feeling of hypoglycemia (or the sensation of a rapid drop in blood sugar) is uncomfortable and anxiety-provoking. It is not unusual for

---

*For those on blood sugar–lowering medication: Aside from taking these precautions, make sure those around you know you are diabetic and those closest to you know what to do in an emergency. Carry some glucose tablets, and make sure you wear a diabetes ID to inform anyone trying to help you of your condition should you lose consciousness or have a seizure.

people to overcompensate for low sugar readings by overconsuming sugary food or drink in an effort to make the feeling go away. Overtreatment sends the blood sugar soaring in the opposite direction, and now the person must deal with high readings. Riding the low/high roller coaster is damaging to the body and brain function.

The feelings associated with low blood sugar are feelings of loss of control, and I encourage patients to keep a premeasured hypo-glycemia treatment on hand (in a briefcase, purse, car, or desk drawer). This set amount of carbohydrate would be the go-to choice in the event of hypoglycemia. A portion-controlled treatment that con-tains the exact amount of carbohydrate you should initially take could be a 4 ounce juice box, glucose tabs, or a small can of regular soda This approach is far better than chugging a half gallon of juice or eat-ing four donuts.

Remember that blood sugar does not rise instantaneously; it will take a few minutes for the brain to register normal blood sugar. Ideally, treat the hypoglycemia with the appropriate amount of carbohydrate, wait ten minutes for the carbohydrate to take effect, and retest your sugar. If further treatment is needed, repeat the process. In this way you will normalize your sugar and not end up swinging into high blood sugar.

HOW TIGHT IS TOO TIGHT?

Is there a downside to someone with diabetes keeping blood sugar tar-gets close to normal? Some experts feel that tight control (for those us-ing insulin or diabetes medications to lower blood sugar) can increase the risk for hypoglycemia. By setting the guidelines a bit higher, a per-son may ward off the chance of low blood sugar. (Note that the ADA guidelines are more lenient than the AACE guidelines for blood sugar.)

Severe hypoglycemia (usually considered to be blood sugar under 50 mg/dL) can lead to seizures, coma, or death. I would define severe hypoglycemia as the blood sugar at which a person is unable to inde-pendently treat herself.

Hypoglycemia itself is not usually fatal. What is most dangerous is what might happen if a person experiences severe hypoglycemia and is driving a car, crossing a street, walking down stairs, operating equip-ment, or holding a baby. It is said that some motor vehicle accidents in which a person has "fallen asleep at the wheel" may be caused by a low blood sugar reaction that impaired driving ability. If blood sugar drops low enough, a person might even experience seizures or become unconscious. There appears to be a link between repeated episodes of severe hypoglycemia and an increased potential for brain damage.

CONTROLLED TREATMENT OF HYPOGLYCEMIA

If a person experiences hypoglycemia, the treatment involves ingesting a quick-acting source of easily absorbed carbohydrate.

There are two levels of hypoglycemia: mild/moderate and moderate/severe. The level of hypoglycemia determines how you will treat the low blood sugar reading.

MILD/MODERATE HYPOGLYCEMIA

If blood sugar is 50–70 mg/dL, choose one of the following forms of treatment (each contains about 15 grams of fast-acting carb):

3–4 glucose tablets
6 ounces regular soda (½ can)
1 cup nonfat milk
3 packets (1 tablespoon) of sugar mixed in water
4 ounces full-strength fruit juice
3 teaspoons (1 tablespoon) honey
8 ounces Gatorade

Wait ten minutes, and retest your blood sugar. If blood sugar rises to more than 80, you are back in a normal zone and should eat a meal or snack with appropriate carbs and protein within the next half hour (a half sandwich or individual package of peanut butter crackers should suffice).

If after ten minutes there is no improvement, another 15 grams of fast-acting carbohydrate should be given. Repeat the treatment up to three times. If blood sugar does not rise over 80, call for emergency assistance.

MODERATE/SEVERE HYPOGLYCEMIA

If blood sugar is under 50 mg/dL, the initial treatment must be doubled to contain about 30 grams of rapid-acting carbohydrate:

6–8 glucose tablets
12 ounces regular soda (1 can)
2 cups nonfat milk
6 packets of sugar in water
8 ounces juice
6 teaspoons (2 tablespoons) honey
16 ounces Gatorade

Wait ten minutes, and make sure sugar rises to more than 80. If not, take an additional 15 grams of carbs, wait ten minutes, and retest. If readings don't exceed 80 after three treatments, call emergency services for assistance. .

WHAT DIABETES MEDICATIONS CAN CAUSE LOW BLOOD SUGAR?

Hypoglycemia can occur as a side effect of some diabetes medications, including the following oral diabetes medications that increase insulin production and lead to hypoglycemia (brand name appears in parentheses):

- chlorpropamide (Diabinese)
- glimepiride (Amaryl)
- glipizide (Glucotrol, Glucotrol XL)
- glyburide (DiaBeta, Glynase, Micronase)
- nateglinide (Starlix)
- repaglinide (Prandin)
- sitagliptin (Januvia)
- tolazamide (Tolinase)
- tolbutamide (Orinase).

Certain combination pills can also cause hypoglycemia, including:

- glipizide and metformin (Metaglip)
- glyburide and metformin (Glucovance)
- pioglitazone and glimepiride (Duetact)
- rosiglitazone and glimepiride (Avandaryl)
- sitagliptin and metformin (Janumet).

Certain injectables can cause hypoglycemia, including:

- Byetta
- Symlin
- Victoza
- Insulin.

It is up to the physician and patient to agree upon the tightness of blood sugar control based on the patient's personal health story. Every patient is different, and targets are not written in stone. On one hand, tight control is shown to prevent, forestall, and may even reverse some of the potentially devastating consequences of diabetes. On the other hand, tight control of diabetes for individuals using insulin or certain other diabetic medications may raise the risk of hypoglycemia.

Brenda Becomes Hypoglycemic

When Brenda was diagnosed with type 2 diabetes, it came as no surprise. She had been warned for years that she had borderline diabetes, and in the past three years, the term borderline was replaced with the term prediabetes. Both of Brenda's parents had type 2 diabetes, as did her maternal grandma. She felt it was inevitable that she would be diagnosed, but she was a little put off that she was diagnosed at age 32.

Her diagnosis came during her annual physical. Her lab work showed her fasting glucose was 146 (normal = 65–99 mg/dL). Her doctor then sent her for a hemoglobin A1C (normal = 5.0–5.6%), and Brenda's was 6.9. Her previous glucose was 115 (prediabetes), and her previous A1C was 6.2 (prediabetes).

Brenda's physician prescribed a dose of glyburide (oral medication that lowers blood sugar by prodding the pancreas to release more insulin) to be taken daily before breakfast and dinner. She was prescribed a home blood glucose monitor, and after some practice, she became proficient at self-testing. She was advised to test first thing in the morning and two hours after the start of one meal per day.

Brenda read that glyburide was a medication that would lower her blood sugar. She felt this would be great because high blood sugar was her problem. She followed her diet perfectly but didn't begin to increase activity. She noticed that in short order, diet and medication brought her readings into the normal range.

She realized that exercise (an increase in physical activity of at least thirty minutes over and above her usual day) would spare her muscle and enable her to burn fat. It would also lower her blood sugar and increase her metabolic rate.

The next afternoon, one and a half hours after the start of lunch, she exercised by taking a thirty-minute walk in the spring air. She was surprised at how quickly the time passed. Before she knew it, she was home. She tested her blood sugar and it was . . . down to 82? Wait a minute. Two hours after lunch, and her reading was only 82? Wow . . . this exercise really did help things out.

Later that afternoon, Brenda ate her neutral snack (a handful of almonds and a cheese stick). At about 4:00 PM, she started to feel odd. She was a little light-headed, slightly dizzy, and very hungry. She ate a scoop of cottage cheese and felt no better. She decided to test her blood sugar. Sure enough, her reading was 62.

Brenda realized she was experiencing hypoglycemia. She read that the treatment should be to take ½ cup juice, wait ten minutes, and test again to see that the reading exceeded 80. Sure enough, her reading was now 100. She felt much better.

The same thing happened whenever she exercised. She ended up having to treat low blood sugar sometime in the hours after she finished her workout. She called her physician, who was pleased to reduce her medication.

Now, following her diet and exercise in the Diabetes Miracle lifestyle, she is medication- and hypoglycemia-free. Exercise has taken the place of medication and she has all positive side effects.

MEDICATIONS, INSULIN, AND ALTERNATIVE THERAPIES

A diagnosis of type 2 diabetes does not necessarily mean that you will need to begin taking medication for blood sugar. As you now know, diabetes is a progressive disease. Depending on how long you have actually had diabetes prior to your actual diagnosis, the need for medication may or may not be present.

The first line of treatment often is to make the correct lifestyle changes and ascertain whether these changes can produce normal blood sugar. The diet found in *The Diabetes Miracle*, along with exercise, is what many people with diabetes use to get control of their blood sugar. If after a period of time, your readings are in the normal range—with fasting blood sugar usually less than 110–120 mg/dL, and your two-hour postprandial blood sugar usually less than 140—you can likely manage your type 2 with no medication. (Your doctor can help you to set a time limit to assess if diet and exercise may be adequate for blood sugar control.) If after giving diet and exercise a real trial, your readings do not fall into the normal range, you and your physician can make a decision regarding adding medication to your diabetes regimen.

MEDICATION DOESN'T GIVE A LICENSE TO "CHEAT"

Some people mistakenly believe that by taking medication for diabetes, they will have license to eat whenever and whatever they want. I've heard many patients say, "I'll just take medication and eat whatever I please."

Medication does not replace the need for proper diet and exercise. If needed, medication is prescribed in *addition* to proper diet and exercise. Your medication needs are based on your blood sugar readings. When unhealthy lifestyle choices cause blood sugar readings to skyrocket, the amount of medication required to control blood sugar is greatly increased. So, if you do not manage your lifestyle, you will require higher doses of medication. Most oral medications force the pancreas to work harder and thus fatigue faster. By not modifying your lifestyle, you may be pushing the diabetes train on the fast track to requiring insulin injections.

Many medications for diabetes cause the pancreas to work even harder than it already is. (Remember that one of the causes of type 2 diabetes is inadequate production of insulin because of an overworked and fatigued pancreas.) Most blood sugar–reducing medications force increased insulin production and release from an already overtired pancreas. The use of higher doses of unnecessary medications (required because of incorrect diet choices or lack of activity) tires the pancreas faster. As time passes, your oral medication requirements as well as the number and doses of medications will increase. The more medication required to force blood sugar into the normal range, the greater the risk of side effects from those medications, and the faster the pancreas fatigues. After a period of time, oral medications become less effective, and there will most certainly be the need for insulin injections.

When you see someone with type 2 diabetes eating everything and anything and popping a pill, don't assume they are "getting away with it." Their blood sugar is not under control, they are increasing their risk for complications, their medication requirements are increasing, and they will most likely need insulin injections in the future.

Although medication is helpful if diet and physical activity are not enough, remember that medication for diabetes does not fix the root cause of the problem. Medication artificially lowers the readings. If you eat whatever you want, whenever you want, and remain a couch potato, your blood sugar readings will rise higher than necessary and require increasingly higher doses of medication.

The best course of action is to get on board with a healthy diet and exercise plan that works within your lifestyle. This will provide the backdrop for your best readings. If after adjusting diet and exercise, it is determined that your current medical condition warrants the use of medication for blood glucose control, it does not mean that you have failed. It simply means that at this time, you require medications.

When it comes to prediabetes and type 2 diabetes, medication is just one tool in the arsenal of blood sugar control. Life situations change; medication needs may change as well. Just because you have a diagnosis of diabetes does not mean you require diabetes medication. The dose and type of medication is based upon your blood sugar readings at a particular point in your life. Likewise, if you are prescribed medication for diabetes, don't assume you will require medication forever. Continued blood sugar monitoring will show if and when medication is needed and if and when it needs to be increased, decreased, or possibly eliminated.

Make certain that your physician addresses your medication needs at each visit. Your doses will absolutely need changing from time to time. If you are taking the same dosage and type of medication after ten years of diabetes, something is probably not right. Being complacent doesn't mean things are under control—it can just mean that someone is not reevaluating your medication needs. It's no mystery if you need to change your lifestyle, medication, medication placement, or dosage because the answers are in black and white in your fasting glucose, hemoglobin A1C, and home blood glucose log book.

ORAL DIABETES MEDICATIONS

People with type 2 diabetes can use oral diabetes medications, whereas those with type 1 diabetes are insulin-dependent—meaning their pancreas can no longer produce insulin, no matter how much oral medication is taken. The only treatment for type 1 diabetes is insulin.

Oral diabetes medications come in different classes and work in different ways. Certain medications work better for certain situations. For example: People with high fasting blood glucose readings but normal post-meal readings will require different medication than people who have normal fasting readings but elevated post-meal readings.

There are four main mechanisms of action for oral diabetes medications:

1. Stimulate the pancreas to produce and release more insulin. Blood sugar doesn't magically decrease when you take a pill; the pill causes the pancreas to release more insulin, which in turn attaches to insulin receptors on your fat and muscle cells and enables excess sugar to enter the opened cells (primarily fat cells).
2. Decrease the release of glycogen from the liver. These medications don't actually shuttle blood sugar into cells; rather, they suppress the liver from depositing excess sugar into the bloodstream.
3. Block the stomach enzymes that break down carbohydrates into blood sugar. Carbohydrates then pass undigested through the GI tract without converting into blood sugar.
4. Increase the secretion of insulin when blood sugar rises and decrease the release of glycogen from the liver (combination

medications). Many people with diabetes require help with both their fasting and their after-meal readings.

There are currently several classes of oral medications and non-insulin injectables in the United States. These classes work in different ways to lower blood sugar. Sometimes diabetes management requires the use of more than one class of medication. The classes are as follows:

1. Sulfonylureas
2. Meglitinides
3. Biguanides
4. Thiazolidinediones
5. Alpha-Glucosidase Inhibitors
6. DPP-4 inhibitors

SULFONYLUREAS

Some medications in this class include (brand names appear in parentheses):

Chlorpropamide (Diabinese)
Glipizide (Glucotrol, Glucotrol XL)
Glyburide (Micronase, Glynase, DiaBeta)
Glimiperide (Amaryl).

Sulfonylureas stimulate the beta cells of the pancreas to release more insulin. Older generations of these medications have been in use since the 1950s. They are usually taken before a meal because they prompt the pancreas to release extra insulin for meal time. If prescribed once a day, they are usually taken right before breakfast; for twice a day dosage, they are usually taken before breakfast and dinner. If taken in excess of the patient's needs, this class of drugs can cause hypoglycemia. Skipping or delaying meals when taking these medications also can cause unhealthy low blood sugar.

All sulfonylurea drugs have similar effects on blood glucose levels, but they differ in side effects, how often they are taken, and interactions with other drugs. Sulfonylureas can help decrease hemoglobin A1C by 1–2 percent. Some possible side effects include hypoglycemia, stomach upset, skin rash/itching, and weight gain.

MEGLITINIDES

Some medications in this class include:
  Repaglinide (Prandin)
  Nateglinide (Starlix).

Like sulfonylureas, meglitinides stimulate the beta cells to release insulin. These drugs are usually taken before each of three meals. Usually, if you must skip a meal, your physician will tell you to skip taking Prandin or Starlix for that mealtime because you might experience hypoglycemia if you take the medication to lower blood sugar and don't eat.

BIGUANIDES

Some medications in this class include:
  Metformin (Glucophage, Glucophage XR, Riomet, Fortamet, and
    Glumetza)

Biguanides lower blood sugar by decreasing the liver's release of glycogen and by improving your muscle receptors' sensitivity to insulin (thus permitting more efficient glucose uptake from the bloodstream). Biguanides do not prompt the pancreas to produce more insulin and do not usually cause hypoglycemia. Possible side effects include diarrhea, bloating, GI upset, and metallic taste in the mouth, so many physicians will start at a low dose and gradually increase it to the required amount. Take metformin with a meal or food. It can be prescribed to take once or twice a day. These drugs can help decrease hemoglobin A1C by 1–2 percent.*

THIAZOLIDINEDIONES

Some medications in this class include:
Rosiglitazone (Avandia)
Pioglitazone (Actos).

The mechanism of action for thiazolidinediones is to help insulin connect better to cells and to reduce liver production of glucose. The first drug released in this class, traglitizone (Rezulin), was found to cause serious liver problems and was subsequently removed from the market. As a result of this finding, liver function tests are recommended before beginning and periodically while you are on this class of drugs. Both Avandia and Actos appear to increase the risk for heart failure in certain individuals. They can be taken independent of food, should be taken at about the same time daily, and do not directly cause hypoglycemia. These drugs can help decrease hemoglobin A1C by 1–2 percent. In addition to problems with your liver, other possible side effects include respiratory infection, headache, and fluid retention.

ALPHA-GLUCOSIDASE INHIBITORS

Medications in this class include:
Acarbose (Precose)
Miglitol (Glyset)
Voglibose (Volix).

---

*If you are having a medical test that requires the use of dye, or you are having surgery, inform your physician or surgeon that you take metformin. You will most likely be advised to stop taking this medication a day or so before the test or surgery. Your metformin will probably be restarted after the surgery, when you are back to eating and your kidneys are working normally, or forty-eight hours after the dye-related test.

BANNED MEDS

In May 2011, The U.S. Food and Drug Administration announced that it will restrict the sale of the diabetes drug Avandia in U.S. pharmacies and only allow its use for patients with type 2 diabetes who have exhausted all other medications. These restrictions are in response to data that suggest an elevated risk of stroke, liver damage, primary pulmonary hypertension, increased cholesterol, heart attack, and heart failure. Avandia had already been banned in Europe.

In June 2011, Actos was linked to bladder cancer, and a cancer warning will now appear on its label. Its use has been banned in Europe.

The drugs in this class work to block the digestion of starch in foods, such as bread, potatoes, and rice, and to slow the breakdown of simple sugar. Their mechanism of action is to slow the rise in blood sugar after a meal. The medication must be taken with the first bite of the meal so carbohydrates will pass undigested through the GI tract. These medications are known to cause gas, bloating, flatulence, and diarrhea in most people as the undigested carb begins to ferment in the GI tract.

DPP-4 INHIBITORS

Some medications in this class include:

Sitagliptin (Januvia)

Saxagliptin (Onglyza)

Linagliptin (Tradjenta

Combinations: Kombiglyze (Saxagliptin + Metformin),

 Janumet (Sitagliptin + Meformin).

This is a new class of oral medication in the diabetes arsenal. The mechanism of action is to increase insulin secretion when blood sugar levels are high and to signal the liver to stop producing excess amounts of sugar. They can drop HbA1C by 0.70–1.2 percent. They seem to promote less hypoglycemia than the sulfonylureas.

THE HIGH COST OF ORAL MEDICATIONS

Now that you realize the different ways that diabetes medication works, it becomes obvious that the data you provide to your doctor from home glucose testing is integral in determining the help you might need from prescription drugs. Your blood sugar readings will clearly indicate the type, strength, and possible combinations of medications that would be most effective for you.

Some physicians prefer to use combination oral medication therapy to attack the blood sugar problem from different angles. Many people take a sulfonylurea to stimulate insulin production along with a biguanide to decrease the liver's release of glycogen. It is also possible to use a combination of diet, exercise, oral medication, and insulin for type 2 diabetes.

Costs of diabetes medications and supplies can vary from pharmacy to pharmacy. There are also different costs for different classes of diabetes medications. If you have no prescription program, are on a fixed income, or are overwhelmed with the cost of your medications, remind your physician to prescribe the most cost-effective form of medication therapy. Some pharmaceutical companies offer prescription assistance. There are generics for some sulfonylureas and there is a generic Glucophage (metformin).

Once again, oral diabetes medication does not take the place of a healthy diet and exercise. Medication should be used in addition to diet and exercise. It is vitally important for your long-term health to keep your twenty-four–hour blood glucose in a healthy place, and oral medications are often just the ticket to get you there.

INJECTABLES

In recent years, two types of injectables (injected with a prefilled pen-like device) have been marketed to aid in blood sugar control. Two are formulated for use without insulin (Byetta and Victoza); the other is used in conjunction with insulin injections (Symlin). Neither injectable contains insulin.

GLP-1AGONIST (INCRETIN MIMETICS)

Exenatide (Byetta) and Liraglutide (Victoza). These injectables mimic the function of incretin, a hormone that helps signal the pancreas to make more insulin. They also slow the rate of digestion so that food exits the stomach at a slower rate and resultant glucose will enter the bloodstream more slowly, allowing the pancreas more time to release insulin. The slowed digestion (food literally stays for a longer time in the stomach) makes people feel full longer and may decrease how much food they eat, but some people feel nauseous from the injection. GLP-1 agonists also suppress liver glycogen release. These drugs promote a 0.5–1.0 percent decrease in HbA1C.

Byetta and Victoza are designed to use in combination with oral medications. Although injected, they are not insulin and should not be taken with insulin. They are not for use in those with type 1 diabetes. Byetta is injected twice a day within an hour of breakfast and dinner while Victoza is injected at anytime of the day (be consistent) and need not be taken with food.

AMYLIN AGONIST

Pramlintide (Symlin). This is the synthetic version of the human hormone amylin, which is normally produced by the beta cells of the pancreas and released at the same time insulin is released. It helps lower blood sugar levels. The injectable Symlin is used by those who take insulin to get even tighter blood sugar control. Because it can increase the risk of extreme hypoglycemia, patients are carefully selected and monitored closely by their physicians. Symlin is injected prior to major meals with more than 30 grams carbohydrate.

This class of injectables can cause severe hypoglycemia in people with type 1 diabetes. It slows gastric emptying, suppresses liver release of insulin, and maintains a feeling of fullness (as food remains in the stomach longer), and nausea may occur.

THE "I" WORD: INSULIN

When diet and physical activity are not enough, and if oral medications are no longer effective or are not appropriate based on other medical conditions, insulin injections may be the medication of choice for blood sugar control. An example of a case in which oral meds might be contraindicated would be if a person develops a kidney disorder and his oral medications would normally clear his body through his kidneys. His physician will most likely change his medication from oral medication to insulin.

As you know, the hormone insulin is involved in the metabolism of carbohydrates. The case of insulin and people with type 2 diabetes is different from those with type 1 diabetes. People with type 1 diabetes make little to no insulin and must take insulin to maintain life. Type 2's may actually have more circulating insulin than someone without diabetes. After years of excess insulin release and increasing insulin resistance (a state that leaves insulin receptors misshapen and less effective), the pancreas fatigues and is no longer able to produce the amount of insulin that is needed to get the job done. Higher-than-normal sugar accumulates in the bloodstream but cannot enter the cells efficiently. If the pancreas fatigues to the point that oral medications can no longer stimulate its release (beta cell fatigue), a person with type 2 diabetes can require insulin injections to take up the slack.

THE SOURCE OF COMMERCIAL INSULIN

Insulin was discovered in the 1920s. Prior to this time, people who developed type 1 diabetes did not survive. The first successful insulin used in humans came from the pancreases of cows and later from pigs. Animal-based insulin was purified, bottled, and sold. Although this insulin was effective and became a lifesaver for those with type 1 diabetes, some people developed allergies to the foreign protein it contained. It took until the 1980s for technology to create artificial insulin that mimicked human insulin. Lab-engineered insulin is far less allergenic and has greater stability and reliability.

Insulin cannot be taken in pill form or by mouth because it is composed of protein and would be digested like a protein-containing food.

TYPES OF INSULIN FOR DIABETES TREATMENT

Although all insulin is a hormone that enables blood sugar to enter cells, there are many types of insulin used to treat diabetes. They are classified by how soon after injection they begin to work and how long their effects last.

Rapid-Acting (Humalog, NovoLog, Apidra). May be injected or used in insulin pumps. This type of insulin works almost immediately to quickly reduce blood sugar. It is used to control blood sugar from meals or to correct a high blood sugar number that exists before a person even eats a meal. Rapid-acting insulin is injected at the time of the meal because it begins to work almost immediately, within the first ten to fifteen minutes. Rapid-acting insulin does its job to lower blood sugar and then is spent. It is often used in combination with intermediate or long-acting insulin.

Short-Acting (Regular R). This type of insulin also is used to control blood sugar from meals but takes a bit longer to kick in. It is injected about thirty minutes prior to mealtime because it takes up to an hour to work. It is often used in combination with intermediate or long-acting insulin.

Intermediate-Acting (NPH or Lente). One injection of an intermediate-acting insulin can control blood sugar for half the day or overnight. After intermediate insulin is injected, it takes hours to reach peak effectiveness; however, it provides longer duration than rapid- or short-acting insulin. Intermediate-action insulin is often used to control blood sugar from food as well as sugar from the liver's release between meals and overnight. Intermediates can be used in combination with rapid- or short-acting insulin or are sometimes used at night as an adjunct to oral medications used during the day. Because they have a peak time—a time when they reach their highest strength—meals must be eaten on time, or hypoglycemia may result.

Long-Acting (Lantus, Levemir, Ultralente). One injection of long-acting insulin controls baseline blood sugar for almost a full day (almost twenty-four hours). Not typically used to cover blood sugar resulting from meals, long-acting insulin is usually used to help control sugar from the liver's release between meals and overnight. Long-acting insulin is often used in combination with rapid- or short-acting insulin or as a nighttime-only injection for people who take daytime oral medications.

Premixed (Humulin 70/30, Novolin 70/30, NovoLog 70/30, Humulin 50/50, Humalog 75/25). Premixed insulins contain a combination of intermediate- and rapid- or short-acting insulins. The numbers indicate the percentage of intermediate- and shorter-acting insulin (70/30 insulin is 70 percent intermediate-acting insulin and 30 percent rapid- or short-acting insulin).

Based on your individual situation, your physician will prescribe the best type of insulin for your needs and advise you on when to test your blood sugar and when and how to make adjustments in your insulin program as needed.

STORING INSULIN

Unopened insulin can be stored in the refrigerator or at stable room temperature. Storing the vials/pens on the refrigerator door is not recommended because of greater temperature fluctuations. If unopened, insulin vials or pens will last until their expiration date. Once the vial or pen is opened, insulin can be stored at room temperature or refrigerated and will remain useable for twenty-eight days. It's a good idea to mark the date you opened the vial or pen and make sure to discard any leftover insulin after the twenty-eighth day. Keep your insulin out of bright light and free from wide swings in temperature. Insulin is a protein; it will "cook" and become totally ineffective if exposed to high heat. It will also become ineffective if frozen. The safe temperature range is between 36 and 86 degrees F.

ADMINISTERING INSULIN

Insulin can be administered using three different methods: syringe, insulin pen, and insulin pump.

SYRINGE

Syringes remain the most common method of insulin delivery in the United States, although the use of insulin pens is quickly gaining in popularity. Syringes remain the least expensive method, are easy to use, and are always in stock at pharmacies. If you require two types of insulin (rapid and intermediate), your physician may direct you to combine them in one injection, but some insulin types cannot be combined; you must check with your physician or pharmacist. Most insurance plans cover syringes. Over the years, needles have become thinner and shorter with finer points; they now have lubricated coatings that make them more comfortable to use. All of these features make the process of injecting simpler, more practical, and more pain-free than ever before.

The syringe you use must match your insulin concentration. For example, U-100 syringes must be used with U-100 insulin. (U-100 insulin means there are 100 units per cc of this insulin; it is the most common strength of insulin in the United States.) U-100 syringes come in different sizes. If your total insulin dose requires:

30 units or less, use a 3/10 mL/cc syringe (each line equals 1 unit)
60 units or less, use a ½ mL/cc syringe (each line equals 1 unit)
100 units or less, use a 1 mL/cc syringe (each line equals 2 units).

Reusing syringes is not recommended by the manufacturer because there is a greater risk of infection, contamination, and dulling of the needle that can lead to more painful injections. Never share syringes with anyone because of the possibility of passing blood-borne disease.

INSULIN PEN

The insulin pen is used by more than 90 percent of insulin users in Asia and Europe and is increasing in popularity in the United States. There are two types of pens: durable (the pen is a durable device and insulin cartridges are loaded) and disposable (all-in-one disposable pens). Both have dial-up dosing and are used with disposable screw-on pen needles. Short, thin needles are available. Pens are more convenient, easier to transport and use, give more accurate doses, and are wonderful for the visually impaired. Insurance coverage for those in the United States varies greatly for pens so check with your provider. Each disposable insulin pen contains 300 units of insulin.

Disposing of Syringes, Pen Needles, and Lancets

Many hospitals participate in safe syringe disposal programs for people who use syringes, lancets, or pen needles. For a small fee, they provide a sharps container that gets returned to the facility for disposal when it is filled and a replacement container is provided.

For home disposal, your local pharmacist or waste authority may recommend that you dispose of used sharps in an empty detergent bottle with a screw-on top. Remove the needles from the syringe with a needle cutter (available at a pharmacy). When the container is filled, tape the lid closed with duct tape and label "Medical Waste, Don't Recycle." Discard with household trash (not your recycling).

You might also consider using a destruction device that uses high heat to melt used needles and lancets. Once the used sharp is destroyed in the device, the remaining syringe and melted metal can be disposed of in the garbage (not recycling).

CHOOSING AN INJECTION SITE*

Insulin is injected right under the skin into fatty tissue for better absorption and less sensation. The abdominal area (belly) is the most commonly used site, although insulin can be injected in the back of the upper arm, outer thighs, and even the fatty tissue of the buttocks. The speed of absorption is quickest in the belly area, followed by the back of the upper arm, outer thighs, and finally the buttocks. Don't inject on or near moles, scars, or within a two-inch diameter of the navel (belly button).

Choose a slightly new location for each injection. It is important to rotate sites because overusing one injection site can cause tissue thickening, lumps, and fatty deposits, all of which will decrease insulin's ab-

---

*http://www.uwhealth.org/healthfacts/B_EXTRANET_HEALTH_INFORMATION-FlexMember-Show_Public_HFFY_1105110025928.html.

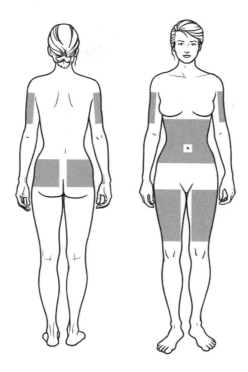

Choosing an Injection Site

sorption. If you always inject in your abdominal area, you should rotate injections around that site.

Another good idea is to give your injections in the same general area at the same time of day. If you take your morning insulin in your abdomen and your evening insulin in your outer thigh fatty tissue, keep it this way consistently, rotating injections within each site area by a little bit each day. This will give your blood sugar readings more stability than using your abdomen one morning, upper arm that night, outer thigh the next morning, and abdomen the next night.

If you intend to exercise, don't inject near the muscles you will be using. For example, if you intend to walk, run, or ride a bike, don't inject insulin in your outer thigh prior to exercise.

How to inject insulin:

1. Wash hands with warm soapy water.
2. Clean the site. Make sure the injection site is clean with soap and water or an alcohol pad. Dry the area. If skin is left wet, you won't be able to ascertain that all the insulin got under the skin.
3. Pinch up a fold of skin surrounding the site you've selected. Hold it firmly with one hand.
4. Insert the needle. Faster is better to minimize sensation; slow insertion is more painful. Try inserting the needle almost like you would toss a dart.
5. Needle angle: For adults or those with ample fatty tissue, insert at a 90-degree angle. Thinner adults may need to inject at a 45-degree angle. Try to get the needle all the way into fatty tissue below the skin, but not so deep that it hits the muscle below.
6. Inject the insulin. Once inserted, push the syringe plunger all the way in with a slow, steady motion, or firmly press the insulin pen injection button. The injection should take a couple of seconds, unless you take a very small dose. (Once the plunger or injection button is pressed, I'd suggest counting to five before removing the needle.) Let go of the skin.
7. Remove the needle by pulling straight out. Twisting or shifting the needle's position will cause pain. Do not rub or massage the skin where the insulin is injected; it can affect how fast the insulin is absorbed and acts within the body.

INSULIN PUMP

Insulin pump therapy is an alternate insulin delivery system that most closely mimics the action of a healthy pancreas. Although insulin pump technology was introduced in the 1970s, it wasn't until the early

1990s that the pump was made practical for users. The insulin pump administers rapid-acting insulin around the clock without your having to give yourself multiple injections.

The pump itself does not monitor your blood sugar or set the program for how much insulin you will receive. Your physician or diabetes educator will work closely with you and use your blood sugar readings to set two rates of insulin: your basal rate and your bolus rate. The basal rate is a very small amount of insulin that is pumped around the clock to match the sugar that is released by the liver between meals and during the night while you sleep. The bolus rate is the amount of insulin needed to correct high readings and for the carbohydrates you will consume at a meal or snack.

The actual pump device is small, about the size of a small cell phone. The pump houses the insulin supply and is worn outside the body. It is usually attached to a belt or waistband, but there are pump accessories that allow for the pump to be "hidden" depending on the clothing you are wearing. Flexible tubing connects the pump to the wearer and is inserted just under the skin into fatty tissue. The tubing is replaced every two to three days. The pump can be disconnected for showering, swimming, or changing clothes. There are also disposable insulin pumps that do not require tubing. The tiny pump is mounted on a disposable skin patch.

If you use an insulin pump, it is important to regularly test your blood glucose often including before meals and at bedtime. Your physician will base your settings on accurate blood sugar readings. The pump is effective as long as you check your blood sugar readings and your pump is programmed with the right settings to match your body. As the pump is a mainly a delivery device for insulin that takes away the need for multiple injections and can help achieve tighter blood sugar control, it is still important to maintain a healthy diet and exercise while using an insulin pump.

ALTERNATIVE THERAPIES FOR DIABETES

Although there are certainly many medication choices available to help control blood sugar, people around the world are seeking alternative therapies to medication.

- Acupuncture has been shown to offer relief from chronic pain and is sometimes used by people suffering from diabetic nerve damage.
- Biofeedback emphasizes relaxation and stress-reduction techniques to help people learn to deal with the body's response to pain (neuropathy).
- Guided imagery is a relaxation technique in which a person thinks of peaceful images or images that foster a sense of control over diabetes.

MINERALS AS THERAPY

Chromium. Usually ingested in the form of chromium picolinate, this mineral has been reported to improve diabetes control by enhancing production of glucose tolerance factor, which has been said to improve the activity of insulin. Most people in the United States are not chromium deficient and get plenty of chromium in the foods they eat, including meat, whole grains, some fruits and vegetables, and even certain spices. Without a chromium deficiency, taking extra chromium will not make a difference in glucose tolerance factor.

Magnesium. A deficiency of magnesium may hamper blood glucose control. Magnesium deficiency interrupts insulin production in the pancreas and increases insulin resistance. There is also evidence that a deficiency may contribute to some diabetes complications. The American Dietetic Association recommends that magnesium supplementation be given only if the patient has magnesium deficiency. The ADA suggests increasing intake of magnesium-containing foods. Legumes, nuts, whole grains, and vegetables will help you meet your daily dietary need for magnesium.

HERBAL REMEDIES

Herbal treatments are not formally recognized by the AMA, ADA, or FDA. However, there is research being conducted, studying the usefulness of herbs in the treatment of diabetes. Just like any other medication or supplement, always remember to report their use to your health care provider for possible interactions with medications.

Pterocarpus marsupium (*Indian kino, malabar kino, pitasara, venga*). This plant has long been used in India as a treatment for diabetes. A flavonoid extracted from the bark of this plant has been used to prevent beta cell damage in rats.

Bitter melon (**Momordica charantia**). Bitter melon, also known as balsam pear, is a tropical vegetable cultivated in Asia, Africa, and South America. It is said to have glucose-lowering ability. There are three primary compounds within bitter melon that seem to help lower blood sugar levels. These compounds include charatin, alkaloids, and peptides.

High doses of bitter melon juice can cause abdominal pain and diarrhea. Small children or anyone with problems regarding hypoglycemic reactions should never take bitter melon because this herb may trigger low blood sugar. Furthermore, people with diabetes taking hypoglycemic drugs or insulin should use bitter melon with caution because it may increase the effectiveness of the drugs, leading to severe hypoglycemia.

Fenugreek (**Trigonella foenum-graecum**). Experimental and clinical studies have demonstrated the antidiabetic properties of fenugreek seeds. The active ingredient of fenugreek is found in defatted fenugreek seed powder. It also has been reported to aid in lowering triglycerides and LDL cholesterol.

Asian ginseng. This root is commonly used in traditional Chinese medicine to treat diabetes. It is reported to enhance pancreatic insulin release and is said to have a direct blood sugar–lowering effect.

Bilberry. This plant has been reported to lower the risk of some diabetic complications, such as cataracts and retinopathy.

Ginkgo biloba. This extract may prove useful for prevention and treatment of early stage diabetic neuropathy and may help support blood vessel health and tone.

Cinnamon. This spice is said to increase cells' sensitivity to insulin. This would help improve the efficiency of insulin and increase the conversion of glucose to energy. Cinnamon is also reported to lower LDL cholesterol and triglycerides. The University of Maryland and the University of Michigan both suggest that supplementation with cinnamon can benefit those with type 1 and type 2 diabetes. A clinical trial that studied only sixty individuals with diabetes concluded that consuming up to 6 grams of cinnamon each day will help regulate blood sugar levels as well as reduce overall cholesterol levels.

POSITIVE AFFIRMATION

I believe in positive affirmation to help control blood sugar, reduce stress, improve mood, and perhaps encourage positive events. Most people realize that there is a running dialogue in the back of their thoughts. Although they don't necessarily talk to themselves or answer their thoughts aloud with their voice, the mind is constantly communicating internally.

A person who listens to an internal channel of negative self-talk begins to believe in the negativity of the situation. A person who is tuned in to positive self-talk usually lives a more positive, productive, forward-moving life. How you react to certain situations is akin to the "glass half empty/glass half full" metaphor. Two people can hear the same news, witness the same event, and encounter the same people but interpret things differently. Some people lean toward the negative, others the positive.

Below is an example of positive self-talk regarding diabetes (I won't give an example of negative self-talk because I don't want to give you any negative ideas about the diagnosis):

I was born with the genetic predisposition to develop type 2 diabetes. I didn't even know I had the possibility of developing it. The road that I traveled from Metabolism B to prediabetes or type 2 diabetes has taken years. During these years, until now unknown to me, my pancreas was overreleasing insulin. Excess insulin made me fatter on the inside (cholesterol/triglycerides) and outside (belly fat).

After years of excess insulin release, my pancreas began to fatigue and slowly but surely produced less insulin. My cells began to resist the insulin I made, and the hormone became less effective. During the time between excess insulin production and less-than-necessary insulin production, I developed fat around my middle, higher LDL cholesterol, higher triglycerides, higher blood pressure, lower vitamin D, and finally higher blood sugar. This metabolic disease has the potential to cause serious complications to my organs, nerves, and blood vessels: This cannot be denied. However, I know this metabolic disease is 100 percent controllable. There is no such thing as diabetes that cannot be controlled!

Before I knew I had diabetes, I took my health for granted. I ate whatever I wanted, whenever I wanted. I didn't exercise because I felt I had more important things to do. I didn't regularly visit my physician and had no idea that my insides (cholesterol, triglycerides, blood pressure, and blood sugar) were out of whack. I was living in the dark and unknowingly causing myself to become sicker — mentally, physically, and emotionally.

Now, with this diagnosis, I have seen the light regarding my wonderful body. I choose to eat in a way that my body can handle. I am physically active for my health and well-being. I see my physician regularly, monitor my own blood sugar, and feel responsible for my good health. I am empowered because I know I can keep this diagnosis under control and actually lead a healthier, happier life because of it.

To treat this condition, I will make the right choices regarding food, exercise, and medication (if needed). My daily blood sugar results will tell me if food and exercise are enough. If they are not, I will use food, exercise, and medication. The dose of medication is correct when, along with my proper diet and exercise, the medication helps to bring my readings into normal range.

Because of this diagnosis, and my full understanding of my metabolism, I finally know who I was, who I am, and where I am going.

In conclusion to this chapter on medication and other treatments for diabetes, I'd like to emphasize that type 2 diabetes has its roots in a genetically mediated hormonal imbalance, and its onset is the result of years of metabolic mayhem.

By testing your blood sugar and working with your doctor, you can determine the best treatment program for you and your own personal condition. Regardless of the treatment — whether it be medication, alternative therapies, positive self-talk, or a combination of all three —

one thing remains certain: The root of diabetes control is in proper diet, exercise, and lifestyle. If normal blood sugar cannot be achieved through natural means, then diet, exercise, and healthy lifestyle remain, and medicinal therapy can be added. Medication never takes the place of a healthy lifestyle . . . it is added to a healthy lifestyle!

Conclusion: Living Well with the Diabetes Miracle Lifestyle

The diagnosis of type 2 diabetes should no longer be considered a life sentence. Your type 2 diabetes did not appear overnight. Those diagnosed with it were born with the genetic propensity to develop the disease, and life's stressors pushed their metabolic makeup further and further down the tracks, from Met B to prediabetes to diabetes.

The positive news is that no matter where you are on the rail line, the Diabetes Miracle can improve and radically change your life and health for the better. Those with Met B can stop their progression to prediabetes. Those with prediabetes can stop the train before they become diabetic and return their engine to the Met B zone. Those who have crossed the line to type 2 diabetes can maintain excellent health on little to no medication without suffering the long-term complications associated with diabetes that is out of control. At the same time your blood sugar is improving, so will your total cholesterol, LDL cholesterol, HDL cholesterol, Vitamin D, hemoglobin A1C, triglycerides, blood pressure, weight, and overall well being!

The study of the human body and how it works (anatomy and physiology) is not a finite science, and we certainly don't know all there is to know about diabetes. The more technologically advanced we become, the more we are able to learn about the miracle of the human body. But technology alone won't give us all the answers if we forget the basics.

I believe that one of the detriments to moving forward in health care has become ultra-specialization and closed-mindedness when it comes to returning to grassroots knowledge of the human body. We no longer always ask the important questions: How does the body work when all is well, and what changes when it is not well? How does normal metabolism work, and what are the differences when a person has a metabolic aberration?

In this era, we have a tendency to view medication as a substance or preparation to treat a disease or illness. We are accustomed to taking medications to treat elevated cholesterol, blood pressure, blood sugar, anxiety, depression, osteoporosis, and most other conditions that ail us.

Note that the medications we are prescribed for diabetes, hypertension, cholesterol, and so on do not cure the conditions; they only temporarily treat the symptoms without getting to the root cause of these health issues. Without medications, the unhealthy readings return, sometimes within hours. Because the root of the problem remains unresolved, our dependence on medication remains.

I am not opposed to taking medication if it is needed, but I feel the first prescription should be lifestyle changes that match the individual's condition and allow a person to naturally correct his course. Remember that every medication has a side effect, and side effects are usually not positive.

I'm fairly certain that in the big picture, humans weren't meant to take pills to force our bodies into the normal range of functioning. Although there are some diseases that do require medication, and certainly medication can be taken for the short term for a temporary illness or disorder, when it comes to many health issues—particularly those that can be slowed or resolved by lifestyle changes—sadly, we've been conditioned to think we can simply take a pill for it and go on with our lives.

The truth is that if we do need medication, we still need to live a healthy lifestyle that matches our body's needs in addition to taking the medicine. There is no such thing as "just take a pill for it" unless you are willing to sacrifice other parts of your body in the process, such as the heavy wear and tear on your liver and kidneys from high doses of medications.

The Diabetes Miracle is the only side effect–free prescription for the bodies of the millions of people born with the genetic predisposition to metabolic syndrome, prediabetes, and type 2 diabetes. It should be the first prescribed medicine. If after making the simple lifestyle changes, a person's health has not returned to normal, a minimal amount of medication can be used in addition to the program to ensure optimal health and well-being.

I wish each and every one of my readers the very best of health, happiness, peace, and well-being. Please help to spread the word of *The Diabetes Miracle*. We can help ourselves and others to get healthy without dependence on pharmaceuticals and expensive tests or procedures. The body is a system of checks and balances, and we now know so much more about the checks and balances of a body with Met B, prediabetes, and type 2 diabetes. The answer is plain, simple, and largely under our control.

Miracles,
Diane

FOR MORE INFORMATION ABOUT DIANE KRESS AND THE DIABETES MIRACLE

www.miracle-ville.com

The official interactive subscription website for followers of Diane Kress' Miracle series, including the Diabetes Miracle and the Metabolism Miracle programs. Features 24/7 live chat, Diane's video blogs, Diane Kress' answers to YOUR personal questions, forums, recipes, tips, news, and positive support. Miracle-Ville is where "Miracles Meet."

BLOGS

www.thediabetesmiracle.com
www.dianekress/wordpress.com
www.themetabolismmiracle.com

TWITTER

Follow Diane on Twitter: @DianeKress.

FACEBOOK

Diane has two groups on Facebook: The Metabolism Miracle and The Metabolism Miracle New Group.

LINKEDIN

Find Diane on LinkedIn: Diane Kress.

DTIME

Visit www.onetouch.com/DTime to watch One Touch's diabetes education series on self-management, featuring Diane Kress. Diane Kress, Diabetes Miracle, and DTime are perfect together!

Acknowledgments

Special thanks to:

Diana Kresefski: Once again, I thank my daughter, assistant, and best friend for all her help managing the private practice, creating, developing, and managing miracle-ville.com, putting out the MANY daily fires while remaining cool under pressure, and for all her help with *The Diabetes Miracle.* I couldn't have devoted the countless hours to this project without you devoting all the time and hours to everything else. You are wise beyond your years and have taught me a thing or two (or three).

Michael Scott Simon, Esq.: Many thanks for all the behind-the-scenes work you have done for the Miracle from Day 1. You have always been a great source of support, and I look forward to working with you as the Miracle series continues. Special thanks this time around for the cover photo. . . . You are a man of many talents! "We may not get there easily . . . but we get there." Onward and upward.

To all those at DaCapo Press/Perseus Books Group: I thank those who have supported me in so many ways as the Miracle series continues. Thanks to John Radziewicz, publisher, for giving my books the company's full support and attention. Thank you, Katie McHugh, executive editor, for having the faith to let me run with this project and giving me the help and support I needed to make it all that it deserved to be. I also am grateful to Lara Hrabota and the publicity team for getting the word out and being so very responsive. Thanks to Kevin Hanover, Lindsey Treibel, and the marketing team for the increased profile of *Metabolism Miracle* and *Metabolism Miracle Cook Book* . . . and now *The Diabetes Miracle*. Thanks also to the sales department for everything you do to make certain the book reaches the readers. Once again, I thank Kärstin Painter, editorial services, for her attention to detail and for turning out such a great product, and a tip of the hat to Melissa Root for her excellent copyediting skills. This has been a very in-depth project, and I am very thankful for having such wonderful support from my publishing house.

Sheila Curry Oakes: Thanks for your time and effort in editing the manuscript and helping to make *The Diabetes Miracle* flow into an enjoyable and understandable read. It was a tremendous undertaking and I thank you! You are very talented, and I am so appreciative of your expertise.

Jay Donnelly: Many thanks for the great job you did on the book's charts and tables. I appreciate the many things you do and I always welcome your special "care packages." Looking forward to your next big project deadline: March 11, 2012!

Tom Panchak and Alice Hsueh: Thank you for working with me to provide quality education for those with diabetes through the launch of the DTime program at www.onetouch.com/dtime. *The Diabetes Miracle* and DTime are perfect together!

Phil Kresefski: Sending very special thanks to my personal "Jim Jupiter:" You kept me walking and talking during this long process, and your extra push helped me to move forward (in many ways). We've been together for a lifetime, and we are always learning something new. XOXO.

Albert Einstein: I thank Einstein for the following quote, an inspiration for *The Metabolism Miracle* and *The Diabetes Miracle*: "Everything should be as simple as it is, but not simpler."

Appendix: Charts for Tracking

My Pedometer Steps per Day

	Monday	Tuesday	Wednesday	Thursday	Friday	Saturday	Sunday	Average Steps/Day
My Goal _____ Steps/Day								
My Goal _____ Steps/Day								
My Goal _____ Steps/Day								
My Goal _____ Steps/Day								
My Goal _____ Steps/Day								
My Goal _____ Steps/Day								
My Goal _____ Steps/Day								
My Goal _____ Steps/Day								

Activity Log
Minimum of 30 minutes, 4 to 5 times a week

In each block, indicate minutes of physical activity over and above your norm.

Monday	Tuesday	Wednesday	Thursday	Friday	Saturday	Sunday

Monday	Tuesday	Wednesday	Thursday	Friday	Saturday	Sunday

Body Measurement and Weight Log

Area Measured	Before Program	Date: ___	Date: ___	Date: ___	Date: ___	Date: ___
Neck						
Chest						
Waistline						
Hips (fullest area)						
Right Thigh						
Left Thigh						
Right Calf (midway between knee and ankle)						
Left Calf (midway between knee and ankle)						
Right Ankle						
Left Ankle						
Right Wrist						
Left Wrist						
Right Upper Arm (midway between elbow and shoulder)						
Left Upper Arm (midway between elbow and shoulder)						
Weight						

Total Inches Lost after each 8 week interval					
Total Pounds Lost after each 8 week interval					

Check Sheet for Step 1

Place a check mark next to completed tasks

	Monday	Tuesday	Wednesday	Thursday	Friday	Saturday	Sunday
Liberal Neutral Food Intake							
5 gram Counter - Breakfast							
5 gram Counter - Lunch							
5 gram Counter - Dinner							
5 gram Counter - Bedtime							
5 gram Counter - Middle of the night							
64 oz decaf fluid or water							
AM Vitamins							
PM Vitamins							
Green Tea (2 tea bags)							
Over 30 minutes of exercise							
Fasting Blood Sugar (if applicable)							
Post-Meal Blood Sugar (if applicable)							
Pre-Meal Blood Sugar (insulin users)							

Check Sheet for Step 2

	Monday	Tuesday	Wednesday	Thursday	Friday	Saturday	Sunday
Liberal Intake of Neutral Foods							
11 – 20 Gram carb dam at all meals							
11 – 20 Gram carb snack between meals that exceed 5 hours							
(make sure first carb dam within one hour of wake-up)							
(make sure last carb dam within one hour of bedtime)							
11 – 20 Gram carb dam if awake in the middle of the night							
64 oz decaf fluid or water							
AM Vitamins							
PM Vitamins							
Green Tea 1 bag or 2 bags							
Over 30 minutes of exercise							
Fasting Blood Sugar (if applicable)							
One post-meal reading done if diet +/- oral medication							
Pre-meal and bedtime readings (if on insulin)							
Check (√) if very high stress day							
Check (√) if in pain above your normal pain level							
Check (√) if ill							

Check Sheet for Step 3

Minimum dam = 1 carb serving and Maximum dam = 4 carb servings

Day 1	Time	# of Carb Servings
Wake Up		
Breakfast		
Snack		
Lunch		
Snack		
Dinner		
Bedtime		
Middle of the Night (if applicable)		

	Check (√) if applicable
64 oz decaf fluid or water	
AM Vitamins	
PM Vitamins	
Green Tea 1 bag or 2 bags	
Over 30 minutes of exercise	
Fasting Blood Sugar	
One post-meal reading done if diet +/- oral medication	
Pre-meal and bedtime readings (if on insulin)	
Check (√) if very high stress day	
Check (√) if in pain above your normal pain level	
Check (√) if ill	

Day 2	Time	# of Carb Servings
Wake Up		
Breakfast		
Snack		
Lunch		
Snack		
Dinner		
Bedtime		
Middle of the Night (if applicable)		

	Check (√) if applicable
64 oz decaf fluid or water	
AM Vitamins	
PM Vitamins	
Green Tea 1 bag or 2 bags	
Over 30 minutes of exercise	
Fasting Blood Sugar	
One post-meal reading done if diet +/- oral medication	
Pre-meal and bedtime readings (if on insulin)	
Check (√) if very high stress day	
Check (√) if in pain above your normal pain level	
Check (√) if ill	

Day 4	Time	# of Carb Servings
Wake Up		
Breakfast		
Snack		
Lunch		
Snack		
Dinner		
Bedtime		
Middle of the Night (if applicable)		

	Check (√) if applicable
64 oz decaf fluid or water	
AM Vitamins	
PM Vitamins	
Green Tea 1 bag or 2 bags	
Over 30 minutes of exercise	
Fasting Blood Sugar	
One post-meal reading done if diet +/- oral medication	
Pre-meal and bedtime readings (if on insulin)	
Check (√) if very high stress day	
Check (√) if in pain above your normal pain level	
Check (√) if ill	

Day 5	Time	# of Carb Servings
Wake Up		
Breakfast		
Snack		
Lunch		
Snack		
Dinner		
Bedtime		
Middle of the Night (if applicable)		

	Check (√) if applicable
64 oz decaf fluid or water	
AM Vitamins	
PM Vitamins	
Green Tea 1 bag or 2 bags	
Over 30 minutes of exercise	
Fasting Blood Sugar	
One post-meal reading done if diet +/- oral medication	
Pre-meal and bedtime readings (if on insulin)	
Check (√) if very high stress day	
Check (√) if in pain above your normal pain level	
Check (√) if ill	

Day 3	Time	# of Carb Servings
Wake Up		
Breakfast		
Snack		
Lunch		
Snack		
Dinner		
Bedtime		
Middle of the Night (if applicable)		

	Check (√) if applicable
64 oz decaf fluid or water	
AM Vitamins	
PM Vitamins	
Green Tea 1 bag or 2 bags	
Over 30 minutes of exercise	
Fasting Blood Sugar	
One post-meal reading done if diet +/- oral medication	
Pre-meal and bedtime readings (if on insulin)	
Check (√) if very high stress day	
Check (√) if in pain above your normal pain level	
Check (√) if ill	

Day 6	Time	# of Carb Servings
Wake Up		
Breakfast		
Snack		
Lunch		
Snack		
Dinner		
Bedtime		
Middle of the Night (if applicable)		

	Check (√) if applicable
64 oz decaf fluid or water	
AM Vitamins	
PM Vitamins	
Green Tea 1 bag or 2 bags	
Over 30 minutes of exercise	
Fasting Blood Sugar	
One post-meal reading done if diet +/- oral medication	
Pre-meal and bedtime readings (if on insulin)	
Check (√) if very high stress day	
Check (√) if in pain above your normal pain level	
Check (√) if ill	

My Progress: Fasting Labs, Clothing Size, Medications/Doses

Fasting Labs	Before Program Date ___	Date ___	Date ___	Date ___	Date ___	Date ___
Glucose						
Total Cholesterol						
LDL Cholesterol						
HDL Cholesterol						
Triglycerides						
Hemoglobin A1C						
Vitamin D						
Fasting Insulin						
TSH						
CRP						
Clothing Size (if applicable)						
Shirt Size						
Pants Size						
Dress Size						
Neck Size						
Medications & Doses (Include Supplements)						

Blood Glucose Log for Diet Alone or Diet and Oral Medications

Date	Fasting BG Reading	Post-Meal BG Reading *		
	BG Reading	Name of Meal	# of Hours From Start of Meal	BG Reading

* Indicate: B = Breakfast   BG = Blood Glucose
          L = Lunch
          D = Dinner

Blood Glucose Log for Insulin Users

Date	Pre-Breakfast (fasting)			Pre-Lunch		
	Time	BG	Insulin Units	Time	BG	Insulin Units

Date	Time	BG	Insulin Units	Time	BG	Insulin Units

Date	Time	BG	Insulin Units	Time	BG	Insulin Units

Date	Time	BG	Insulin Units	Time	BG	Insulin Units

Date	Time	BG	Insulin Units	Time	BG	Insulin Units

Pre-Dinner			Bedtime			Hypoglycemia (if applicable)		
Time	BG	Insulin Units	Time	BG	Insulin Units	Time	BG	Treatment

Time	BG	Insulin Units	Time	BG	Insulin Units	Time	BG	Treatment

Time	BG	Insulin Units	Time	BG	Insulin Units	Time	BG	Treatment

Time	BG	Insulin Units	Time	BG	Insulin Units	Time	BG	Treatment

Time	BG	Insulin Units	Time	BG	Insulin Units	Time	BG	Treatment

Index